Bibliotherapy—The Interactive Process: A Handbook

We gratefully acknowledge Hilary Daley-Hynes's rendering of a drawing by an unknown artist. It evokes for us the transforming beauty of the bibliotherapy process.

About the Book and Authors

The recognition that literature can be a healing tool is as old as Aristotle's discussion of catharsis. In bibliotherapy an individual reads or listens to a work of literature specifically for its therapeutic value. But until now a real professional tool was lacking. This handbook, the first of its kind, is designed to teach both professionals and laypersons how to use the whole spectrum of literature—from poetry to science fiction—to promote greater self-knowledge, to renew the spirit, and, in general, to aid in the healing process.

Beginning with an explanation of the theoretical basis for bibliotherapy, the authors then provide a comprehensive overview of the procedures and goals of the discipline. The material is presented in such a way that the process may be adapted to the particular educational or psychological approach favored by the practitioner for the therapeutic treatment of individuals who have been abused or are chemically dependent, physically disabled, emotionally disturbed, hospitalized, in correctional institutions, or simply facing difficult or stressful life situations. The authors also offer insights for using bibliotherapy to promote the healthy growth and development of children and to provide psychological help and guidance to adults and the aging. Case studies from practice and training experiences illustrate the principles of bibliotherapy; in addition, the authors include end-of-chapter study questions for persons involved in therapy and self-help and practicum guides for professionals. Taken together, these materials comprise a unique and invaluable reference work in a new and significant field.

Arleen Hynes, O.S.B., established the first hospital-based training program in bibliotherapy in 1974 at St. Elizabeths in Washington, D.C. **Dr. Mary Hynes-Berry** is a professional writer.

All high poetry is infinite; it is as the first acorn, which contained all oaks potentially. Veil after veil may be undrawn, and the inmost naked beauty of the meaning never exposed.

—Shelley

BIBLIOTHERAPY
The Interactive Process

A Handbook

Arleen McCarty Hynes
and
Mary Hynes-Berry

Routledge
Taylor & Francis Group
LONDON AND NEW YORK

First published 1986 by Westview Press, Inc.

Published 2018 by Routledge
52 Vanderbilt Avenue, New York, NY 10017
2 Park Square, Milton Park, Abingdon, Oxon OX14 4RN

Routledge is an imprint of the Taylor & Francis Group, an informa business

Library of Congress Cataloging-in-Publication Data
Hynes, Arleen McCarty.
Bibliotherapy—the interactive process.
Bibliography: p.
Includes index.
1. Bibliotherapy. I. Hynes-Berry, Mary. II. Title.
RC489.B48H96 1986 615.8'516 86-1582
ISBN 13: 978-0-367-02215-0 (hbk)
ISBN 13: 978-0-367-17202-2 (pbk)

Contents

Tables and Figures

Tables

Figures

Acknowledgments

No one writes a book alone. We all respond to insights from our experiences and gain encouragement in ways we can never fully acknowledge. Yet it is clear that we could never have completed this book without the support of our families to whom our work is dedicated.

We can mention only a few of the many others who contributed to this handbook. Major credit goes to Kenneth Gorelick, M.D., and Rosalie Brown, bibliotherapist, who were Arleen Hynes's colleagues at St. Elizabeths Hospital in Washington, D.C., where they all worked together to develop bibliotherapy as a part of the treatment program and to establish the ongoing training program.

It would not be possible to name the many others at St. Elizabeths who refined our understanding of the bibliotherapeutic process. The superintendents, the psychotherapists who worked with the trainees, the staff, and the patients all played vital roles. But we are especially grateful to Fred Depp, Ph.D., Harriet Murphy, Ph.D., and Elaine Apostles, Ph.D., who gave great encouragement and assisted in research essential to developing the list of strengths discussed in Chapter 11.

We also owe much to certain persons not affiliated with St. Elizabeths. Gerald May, M.D., provided chapter-by-chapter encouragement and suggestions. The careful and discriminating reading of Barbara Allen added the insights of a current worker in developmental bibliotherapy. Joseph Wholey, Ph.D., and Beth Barrett, R.N., both provided expert evaluations that were invaluable in drawing up the record forms. Rhea Rubin and Clara Lack gave warm support throughout the project.

We are deeply grateful for the support of Prioress Sister Evin Rademacher and Sister Katherine Howard of the Benedictine community, who encouraged pursuit of this book. Sister Judith Schaffer and Sister Mary Patrick Murray each helped in specific ways, and Sister Romaine Theisen patiently typed several drafts.

We are also grateful for permission from the authors to use the text of "Eve to Cain" by F. W. Willette and "February" by Peggy Patrick Miles.

Finally, Fred Praeger, our publisher, deserves special thanks for his concern for the people who will benefit from bibliotherapy; if he had not asked that this book be written, it would never have been done.

Arleen McCarty Hynes
Mary Hynes-Berry

Introduction: A Reader's Guide

In Cracow, a rabbi dreamt three times that an angel told him to go to Livovna and that in front of the palace there, near a bridge, he would find a treasure. When the rabbi arrived in Livovna, he told his story to a sentinel, who told him that he, too, had had a dream in which he was told to go to a rabbi's house in Cracow, where a treasure was buried in front of the fireplace. So the rabbi went home and dug at his fireplace and found the treasure.

THE MESSAGE OF THIS EIGHTEENTH-CENTURY Hasidic tale is timeless: Even though you often must seek among others to find it, your spiritual treasure lies within your own heart. As Mircea Eliade said, "To find yourself, you must go to a stranger." In many ways, the tale sums up the essence of bibliotherapy. The *stranger* is the literature we use as the primary tool; the *other* is the bibliotherapist who, with yet *others* (participants in the bibliotherapy group), facilitates the search for the *treasure*—true self-knowledge. We constantly refer to the triad of the literature, the facilitator, and the participant.

Use of the Handbook

This handbook, a practical guide, is addressed primarily to the bibliotherapy facilitator. In it we begin with a descriptive definition of the field and then explore the dynamics of the bibliotherapeutic process and the goals that the process is meant to further. We next examine in turn each of the three major components, beginning with the literature, moving on to the facilitator, and turning finally to the participant. Each part begins with a chapter devoted to the dynamics brought into play by the element of the basic triad under discussion, and the rest of each part is devoted to related strategies and procedures. All chapters open with a vignette that is meant to bring to life the theory or procedure about to be analyzed.

The handbook and the suggestions for training contained in it are based on seven essential components of bibliotherapy formulated by Arleen Hynes and Kenneth Gorelick in 1977-1978, based on their experience at St. Elizabeths Hospital (Hynes 1978c).

1. Didactic information about theories in bibliotherapy, including the differences between clinical and developmental modes, and about mental health outlooks
2. Orientation to a basic humanistic therapeutic outlook
3. Knowledge about and observations of group dynamics
4. Experience in conducting patient-member bibliotherapy sessions and in carrying out the details of professional work such as cooperation with other staff members, writing reports for bibliotherapy supervisors, and entering observations on the patient's records
5. Taking part in group supervision, in which several trainees discuss their reactions to leading groups under the guidance of a psychiatrist or psychologist
6. Professional supervision for each group worked with
7. Experience in a developmental bibliotherapy group made up of fellow trainees

These same components are being considered by the committee of the National Federation of Biblio/Poetry Therapy that is studying standardization for training and certification (Reiter 1978a, 1978b; Lerner 1979).

This handbook is designed for classroom use, for in-service training of practicing mental-health professionals, and for private study by librarians, teachers, nurses, occupational and creative therapists, and any interested lay persons. Instructors for academic or in-service training programs will use the material in this book in accordance with their overall objectives for the class.

We recommend that those who are planning to carry out a self-study program follow certain procedures.

1. If you do not have a mental-health background or experience with bibliotherapy, you will need to find a mental-health professional to supervise your studies. The supervisor can be a psychologist, a psychiatrist, a social worker, a psychiatric nurse, a counselor, or a pastor with professional counseling training. A supervisor who has not practiced bibliotherapy must be willing to read the professional literature on bibliotherapy and poetry therapy to see how this mode differs from his or her professional thrust. These differences will have to be taken into account both when discussing

handbook material and, later, when your performance with a group is being critiqued.

2. You should go carefully through the material a first time before actually beginning to work with participants, discussing the content of the chapters as well as the study guide material with the supervisor.

3. Arrangements should be made to begin doing bibliotherapy with a group, under supervision. Some trainees will have begun this self-study intending to work with a specific population. Others may have to investigate local mental-health programs to find a group. The supervisor may be of assistance in both cases, in the designing and establishment of a suitable training situation.

4. You should plan to work through the handbook a second time—specifically, when you begin conducting a group or working with clients under supervision. The supervisor may want to schedule further discussion of individual chapters, emphasizing issues that have come up in the actual sessions.

5. Those who come to bibliotherapy from outside the mental-health professions must arrange to take academic classes in therapeutic theory and communication, as well as in group theory and dynamics. Clinical bibliotherapists need to take classes that will familiarize them with the major types of mental illness. Those without a strong background in literature will find literature classes and/or library-school courses in reference materials to be of great value.

6. For purposes of eventual certification, you should keep a complete record of (1) contact hours leading groups, (2) contact hours with supervisors or in training workshops, and (3) transcripts of any classes taken to improve understanding of mental-health work or bibliotherapeutic materials.

Because experiential learning will add significantly to your understanding of how bibliotherapy works, we strongly recommend that some arrangement be made to hold a developmental bibliotherapy group concurrently with study of this handbook. Such sessions may occasionally conclude with a critique, but group members should fully engage themselves as *participants,* not merely as observers. The possibility of role confusion will be lessened by having someone other than the classroom teacher or trainer act as the facilitator for the experiential component.

Once actual training with a group begins, tapes or videotapes of the sessions should be used for critiquing whenever possible. If necessary, consult Berger's (1978) book-length treatment of the rationale and techniques involved in using videotapes for psychiatric training. Kenny (1982) also briefly reviews some important points about audiovisuals in the mental-health field.

At the same time, it is critical that you begin keeping records such as those found in Appendix B. In Chapter 11, we have suggested other tools for recording what takes place. Note that the charts are meant neither to supplant the basic written record for each session nor to be used from the very beginning of the training experience. We encourage trainees to gradually begin using the different instruments, one at a time, in the order in which they are presented in the text. In addition, we have found that it is necessary to work with at least two populations in different settings to fully understand how to use and to benefit from the charts concerned with participants' responses. After training is completed, all of these forms are to be used with your bibliotherapy groups.

Materials for Training and Practice

"Study Questions," "Practicum," and "Further Readings" follow each chapter. The study questions involve a rather intensive amount of work. Answering them will not only call upon your understanding of the important issues raised in the chapter but, at times, will also require some outside reading.

The practicum suggestions are equally demanding. They are intended to help you translate an intellectual grasp of bibliotherapy into practice. Both the study questions and the practicum suggestions will direct you to those experiences we have found to be most beneficial in the training programs we have conducted. Important clarification often takes place when class members share and discuss the similarities and differences among their individual responses to the questions or group situations. We strongly urge that the questions and practicum be part of the overall study of bibliotherapy.

The lists of further readings may be most helpful to those who are new to the helping professions. However, persons with some mental-health background and training will find it useful to adapt the general mental-health materials specifically to the relatively new field of bibliotherapy.

Note that the basic bibliography of bibliotherapeutic literature is not extensive, even though it includes materials from the closely related field of poetry therapy. Lerner's articles (1981, 1982, 1984a, and 1984b) are useful, succinct surveys of what is included in the field of biblio/poetry therapy. But we also anticipate that the users of this handbook will familiarize themselves with the books by Rubin (1978a and 1978b), Leedy (1969 and 1973), Lerner (1978), and Schloss (1976). Thus, few specific citations are made to these texts in the reading lists. However, we urge bibliotherapists in training to reread these materials for further insights as they gain experience in the field.

Supplementary Materials

The function of the six *Listening Exercises* in Appendix A is described in Chapter 1. The exercises themselves should be worked through at periodic intervals; for example, we suggest doing one such exercise in conjunction with the study material following each of the first six chapters.

Appendix B includes (1) a form for the chronological record of bibliotherapy sessions conducted, (2) a sample report on bibliotherapy groups, and (3) a form on which to periodically assess your own facilitative skills. It is best that you have this last item filled out several times by a supervisor or some other objective observer as well. The forms may be used as presented or adapted to your specific purposes.

Finally, Appendix C contains a list of the current organizations devoted to bibliotherapy, including addresses and relevant membership information.

The Bibliography of Professional Literature is not meant to be a complete listing of bibliotherapy materials; given space limitations, it includes only professional bibliotherapy and mental-health items that have been directly cited. (Those who do not have access to academic or professional libraries can usually use the interlibrary loan services of their local library to obtain any of these materials.) In addition to professional literature sources, this handbook includes many references to poems, stories, songs, and other items used as bibliotherapeutic material. Unfortunately, the restrictions of space as well as the vagaries of copyright regulations make it impossible to quote more than a few words from most of the works referred to by title in the text. But we do provide bibliographic information about the original source and/or the collection in which a given item can be found; this information is contained in the "Bibliotherapeutic Materials Cited."

— PART 1 —

BASIC UNDERSTANDINGS

1

Interactive Bibliotherapy: A Definition

Chapter 8 of Alexander Solzhenitsyn's Cancer Ward *is an almost perfect introduction to the interactive nature of bibliotherapy.*

Like all the other patients on his ward, Yefrem Podduyev is facing death from cancer. He is very restless and disagreeable until he finds a little blue book from which he reads Tolstoy's story "What Do Men Live By?" The title voices the question that Podduyev finds himself struggling with because of his illness. Using the story as an impetus, he goes around the ward asking everyone that same question. He gets a variety of answers, none of which really satisfies him.

But as he responds to and reflects on these replies, Podduyev comes to a much deeper understanding of Tolstoy's answer—the answer that he wants the others to acknowledge—that men live not by worrying about their own problems but by loving others. After the discussion, Podduyev stops stomping around the ward for hours on end, haranguing the other patients. Instead he lies quietly on his bed, thinking about his past and the meaning of the story.

WE SEE HERE THE INTERACTION of the three key elements in bibliotherapy: Although he is a peer rather than a trained guide, Podduyev acts as a *facilitator;* Tolstoy's story is the *literature;* and the other patients on the ward are the *participants* in this group. At the same time, we see the result of an effective bibliotherapy session. The dialogue about the question posed by the story leads several members of the group to reflect and to arrive at a fresh view of life. In Podduyev's case at least, that insight is internalized and leads to a change in behavior.

The features we have just identified here are found in the working definition of bibliotherapy used in this handbook: "Bibliotherapy uses literature to bring about a therapeutic interaction between participant and facilitator."

Schools of Thought About Bibliotherapy

We should admit from the start that *bibliotherapy* is a somewhat problematic term. If nothing else, the polysyllables are cumbersome, and *bibliotherapy* does not communicate an immediate general impression in the way that the names of other creative therapies, such as art therapy or dance therapy, do.

Nonetheless, this is the term used in many professional indexes. Besides, the etymology is meaningful: *Biblio-* means *books* and, by extension, *literature*; *-therapy* comes from *therapeia*, meaning *to serve* and *to help medically*, and it suggests the concept of healing. Basically, then, bibliotherapy is the use of literature to promote mental health.

This particular capacity of literature to renew and heal the human spirit is at least as old as Aristotle's discussion of catharsis in the *Poetics*. However, *bibliotherapy* should not be considered as an umbrella term for all activities in which books are used for self-improvement. Its use in that way results from confusion (and even disagreement) about exactly where the healing process is centered.

Reading bibliotherapy

One school sees the healing process as taking place through *reading* itself. This mode is a direct development from the traditional role of the librarian as provider of readers' advisory services. In the early 1920s, as an outgrowth of this activity, some librarians made a point of searching out and offering reading materials specifically for their therapeutic potential (Bryan 1939). Since then, numerous librarians, counselors, English teachers, and social workers have compiled lists and made suggestions for reading they believe will help an individual's emotional growth or offer insight into a personal crisis.

In 1949, Caroline Shrodes's dissertation seemed to confirm the definition of bibliotherapy as a process in which an individual reads a book selected specifically for its therapeutic potential for that person. Although her discussion made it clear that the critical interaction was not in the suggestion of the book itself but in how the reader used the content, her definition is still used in some circles to equate bibliotherapy with the process of "prescribing books." We, however, would like to see this activity differentiated as *reading bibliotherapy*.

We do not mean to suggest that recommended readings cannot serve therapeutic ends. On the contrary, there are many cases in which a librarian, teacher, or counselor's thoughtful suggestion has provided a reader with just the right book—a work that triggered a significant and growth-producing feeling-response to some need. The point is that the interaction takes place between the reader and the work and does not directly involve the person who made the suggestion.

Interactive bibliotherapy

We feel it is important that the benefits of the reading process itself not be confused with the distinctive benefits that Shrodes herself suggested would come from discussing the reader's response. Our handbook reflects the thinking behind Rubin's (1978a) and others' recent definitions of bibliotherapy. According to these definitions, there is a significant therapeutic dimension to the facilitated dialogue about the individual's feeling-response to the literature. In other words, in this mode—which can be identified as *interactive bibliotherapy*—the process of growth and healing is centered not as much in the act of reading as in the guided dialogue about the material.

In effect, the triad of participant-literature-facilitator means that there is a dual interaction: The participant's personal response to the story is important, but dialoguing with the facilitator about that response can lead to a whole new dimension of insight. Burt (1972) concisely reviews the literature on this point.

Our emphasis on the therapeutic role served by having feelings clarified in a discussion led by a trained facilitator reflects our understanding that interactive bibliotherapy is more than a potentially healing suggestion—it is a *therapy*. Moreover, we share Jerome Frank's perspective on the nature of therapy:

> Viewed as a healing art rather than as a form of reeducation, the most effective ingredients of psychotherapy lie in those aspects of the therapeutic relationship which raise the patient's morale and inspire him with courage to try new ways of coping with the stresses that beset him. These healing components lie in the realm of feelings. Arousal of such emotions as hope, faith, reverence, even sometimes fear, characterize all forms of healing in nonindustrial societies. Such emotional states seem to increase accessibility to the healer's influence and facilitate attitude change. . . . Proponents of all schools of psychotherapy have always agreed that purely intellectual insight is of little value. (Frank 1972, 110–111)

Thus, in bibliotherapy, the possibility of growth comes from confrontation with genuine feelings. However, raw feeling in itself is not the significant factor. Rather, the beneficial integration that interactive bibliotherapy offers comes from the cognitive process of first *recognizing* feelings and then *sorting out* and *evaluating* the feeling-responses. The process, moreover, is one that is helpful to all—not just to those diagnosed as mentally ill. As T. V. Moore said in discussing his work with adolescents, "The object of bibliotherapy is to supplant impulsive desires by truly human conduct in which one is conscious of the end towards which one is striving, knows what is worthwhile and is determined to attain it" (Moore 1946, 138).

Interactive bibliotherapy and poetry therapy

The recognition that literature can be a formal healing tool reflects a third tradition. In the 1920s, psychiatrist Smiley Blanton, M.D., and his associate, Eli Grieffer, began to propose poetry as a tool that could be used in accordance with a specific methodology. Calling their mode *poetry therapy*, Blanton and Grieffer argued that poems have tremendous potential for use in the diagnosis of important emotional issues; however, they pointed out, it can be difficult—particularly for the emotionally disturbed—to work through such issues unaided. Thus, in poetry therapy an important part of the healing process comes from the communication between therapist and client about how the chosen work bears on the individual's problems and needs (Blanton 1960).

A number of psychotherapy practitioners soon began using creative writing by the client in addition to poems as the basis for both diagnostic and therapeutic sessions (Leedy 1969, 1973; Lerner 1978). We, too, will refer at times to other current therapeutic approaches that use writing, reading, and/or discussion of stories or didactic material but that do not identify themselves as bibliotherapy or poetry therapy.

As the increasing use of the term *biblio/poetry therapy* indicates, poetry therapy and interactive bibliotherapy are synonymous in most critical respects. Both emphasize the importance of the interaction between the triad of participant-literature-facilitator as well as the use of creative writing as material. In this book, however, we use the term *bibliotherapy* because it is generally accepted as a more inclusive term than *poetry therapy*.

Comprehensive Features of Bibliotherapy

Definition of literature

In bibliotherapy the term *literature* is not restricted to poetry or creative writing but, rather, is used in the broadest possible sense. Poetry may be the form used more often than any other; nonetheless, bibliotherapeutic materials encompass not just imaginative but also didactic and informational works. Plays, short stories, novels, essays, magazine articles, and sections from textbooks can all be used in their entirety or in abridged form; so, too, specific passages from any of these forms can be extracted for use.

In fact, the bibliotherapist does not restrict *literature* to the written word. In our world, audiovisuals are an important expression of people's thoughts and feelings. Therefore, recordings, films, videotapes, and filmstrips have all been successfully used as material for bibliotherapy sessions. The added dimensions of sound and/or visual images can increase the impact of language.

Although our definition covers the full spectrum of genres and media, we do feel that all bibliotherapeutic material should involve language and have some internal coherence. Thus, whereas photos, paintings, and music are frequently used to intensify the effect of a written text, of themselves they are not suitable material for a bibliotherapy session. So, too, it will not do to present a group with a list of random words or phrases in order to stimulate free association. We will see that the bibliotherapeutic process depends at least in part on the way the participants relate to a stimulus that has *its own coherence and integrity.*

The facilitator's background and choice of setting

Bibliotherapy facilitators have a wide variety of backgrounds and can choose to operate in two quite different settings. As we have noted, the original poetry therapists primarily used a *one-on-one* relationship between psychotherapist and client. Some poetry therapists and bibliotherapists continue to use this format. However, bibliotherapy is more commonly practiced in a *group* setting.

We refer often to group needs and experiences throughout this book, but the point to remember is that the bibliotherapeutic process and goals function primarily in terms of the individuals who make up the group. By the same token, the facilitator's primary concern is with the needs of the participants *as individuals* rather than with the group as an entity. We will discuss the factors influencing the choice of setting more fully in the context of the bibliotherapist's responsibilities (Chapter 8).

Populations in clinical bibliotherapy

Because the populations that benefit from interactive bibliotherapy are so diverse and because the emphasis necessarily varies from one kind of group to another, practitioners now distinguish between clinical and developmental bibliotherapy. Clinical bibliotherapy is typically one of several creative therapies being used with populations in a specific treatment program. The facilitator is trained to use a psychotherapeutic methodology in which literature acts as the primary tool to help the client(s) toward an integrated personality.

Strategies for dealing with the needs of specific groups will be discussed later, but here we can list the main populations a clinical bibliotherapist might expect to work with.

Emotionally disturbed persons. These clients will be in mental institutions, will be coming back for treatment and follow-up, or will be receiving independent professional treatment. They recognize bibliotherapy as part of their contractual arrangement for therapy. Brown (1977), Crootof (1969), Edgar (1979), Esler (1982), Hynes (1978a, 1978b), Lack (1982), Miller (1978), and Sweeney (1978) describe different hospital programs, whereas Leedy (1969, 1973) and Lerner (1978) detail work with individual patients. Fogle (1980), Mazza and Prescott (1981) and Mazza (1981) indicate the ways in which bibliotherapy has been used as a technique in family therapy.

Clinical bibliotherapy groups are usually formed on the basis of specific populations. For example, one group will be limited to emotionally disturbed adolescents, another to chronically hospitalized patients, and a third to patients who are also suffering from a physical handicap such as blindness or deafness.

Correctional institution residents. Bibliotherapy may be part of a prison program or required as part of probation and parole. Cellini and Young (1976) and Rubin (1974) describe bibliotherapy programs in a prison setting. Norman and Brockmeier (1979) report on the bibliotherapy program developed by Susan Brockmeier for use with youth in a state detention facility in Kearney, Nebraska.

Even though members of this population usually participate under mandate rather than on a voluntary basis, the bibliotherapist will usually insist on the principle that no one can be coerced into revealing personal feelings and insights. The emphasis in prison groups is on helping the participants better recognize and conform to society's norms and standards of behavior. But the bibliotherapist should realize that the participants can also be emotionally unstable and that, in such cases, bibliotherapy may contribute to psychological healing.

Chemically dependent persons. Clinical bibliotherapy groups have been a successful element of institutional drug and alcohol dependency rehabilitation programs (Mazza 1979; Gladding 1979; Goldfield and Lauer 1971; and Schecter 1983). Participants in treatment for dependency are usually intensely involved in self-evaluation and tend to respond effectively to the use of imaginative and informational material as a stimulus for probing their thoughts and feelings.

Populations in developmental bibliotherapy

Developmental bibliotherapy, which has emerged as a way to help all kinds of people in their normal growth and beneficial development, grows out of the recognition that the need to confront personal feelings, to improve self-awareness, and to enhance self-esteem is not confined to mentally ill patients, criminals, or chemically dependent persons. In general, participants in developmental bibliotherapy have specifically chosen this mode to further self-understanding.

Developmental bibliotherapy is typically practiced in groups that have formed and meet in the context of a school, community center, library, church, or synagogue. The basic techniques used to facilitate such groups are the same as those used in clinical bibliotherapy, but the depth of the therapeutic probing differs. At the same time, the bibliotherapist often plays a less active role in the discussion phase than is desirable in clinical groups.

Some of the major populations that have successfully participated in developmental groups include the following.

Adolescents and children. The literature about developmental bibliotherapy is filled with references to programs designed for the young. Schultheis (1969, 1972) is a reading specialist who uses bibliotherapeutically oriented reading and discussion to help build self-esteem among those who need special reading help. Robinson (1980) works with special-education classes in a public library, whereas Frasier and McCannon (1981) use the approach with gifted students. Berg-Cross and Berg-Cross (1976), Jalongo (1983b), and Kenz (1982) give brief overviews and cite books that can be used for bibliotherapy in the classroom, particularly with young children. Zaccaria et al. (1978), Baruth and Phillips (1976), and Benninger and Belli (1982) profile ways in which counselors have used bibliotherapy to help children with behavior problems. Gardner (1969, 1971), a psychotherapist who works with children, has developed a mutual storytelling technique.

Whatever the context, bibliotherapists working with children and adolescents should make it clear that the goals for bibliotherapy are distinct from those of the traditional literature class or reading group. In bibliotherapy, the literature is generally used as a tool to help young people deal with the issues so critical to this stage—self-identity, independence, and self-worth.

Senior citizens. Developmental groups for senior citizens may be organized through a community center, library, church, synagogue, or retirement home. Hynes (1979) gives an overview of the funding and resources involved in working with the aged. Allen and O'Dell (1981) describe how to go about setting up an outreach program for the elderly in the public library; Monroe and Rubin (1983), Neale (1981), Sweeney (1978), Tuzil (1978), and Wedl (1983) discuss working with an institutionalized population. Bresler (1981) gives an account of a specific summer-camp program using creative writing with senior citizens. O'Dell's 1983 article about bibliotherapy is one of several very useful discussions of working with the elderly (see Burnside's 1983 collection). Although Saul and Saul (1974) do not specifically mention bibliotherapy, their article, too, contains an excellent discussion of the benefits of group therapy for patients in a proprietary nursing home and provides valuable insights into working with this population.

In general, the aging have a particular interest in the life-review and evaluation process (Lewis and Butler 1974; Butler 1977; Merriam 1980). But the facilitator should understand that since age is the primary criterion, this population can be extremely diverse. Not only will members of a given group often come from quite different backgrounds, they will also vary both in the need and the ability to cope with such issues as facing personal loss and death, adjusting to a major role change, or coming to terms with diminished physical well-being.

Support groups. Developmental groups established through guidance clinics or vocational guidance centers, as part of an industrial or institutional support program for personnel, or as offshoots from a club or group may focus on issues related to the bonds that members share. For example, a group made up of persons in a retraining program may concentrate on exploring how unemployment affects the individual's self-esteem or alters the way he or she relates to others. Poetry and prayer groups can work specifically on strengthening their spiritual lives. And, in the same way, a Parents Without Partners meeting, a women's awareness group, or a program for battered women might offer bibliotherapy sessions to help members deal with the emotional realities related to their specific difficulties. The possibilities are as unlimited as the reasons underlying the need for mutual support.

Handicapped people. Blind, deaf, crippled, or chronically ill persons can all benefit from bibliotherapy. B. Allen (1981a) discusses such work in the context of disabled people, Brown (1977) discusses the techniques used with physically handicapped and aging persons, Marshall (1981) looks at library work in relation to disabled children, Moody (1964) considers chronically ill people, and Buck and Kramer (1973) describe their work with deaf individuals. In all such cases, the members of a developmental bibliotherapy group can meet as part of a rehabilitation or chronic care program or in a community setting.

Dying patients. Hospice programs look to the emotional as well as the physical needs of terminally ill patients and their loved ones (Butterfield-Picard 1982; Heymann 1974; Pearson 1969). When provided as part of such programs, bibliotherapy can offer patients and their families a meaningful way to deal with the powerful issues and feelings that serious illness raises—specifically, by using literature as a context for discussing concepts and feelings that would otherwise be difficult for patients and family members to bring up.

The bibliotherapist must be sensitive to the special needs of the dying as well as flexible in dealing with them. The length of time either patients or family members can tolerate a bibliotherapy session will vary from individual to individual and will almost certainly change in the course of the illness. Furthermore, dying patients and their families tend to have somewhat different agendas. Hence the facilitator must carefully consider the needs and wishes of all involved in deciding when to work one-on-one with the patient, when to meet separately with family members, and when a session together might help all toward some resolution of relationships before death. Although Reynolds and Kalish (1974) do not discuss bibliotherapy, their article provides important background material for those who plan to work with dying patients in hospital wards.

Public library patrons. Participants who join a developmental group offered through the public library are generally not seeking a clinical therapy session, nor are they likely to share the common bond of age or life situation as do the members of the other groups listed here. But as diverse as the members of a single group may be, they will all likely be interested in using literature to enrich their lives and to enlarge their view about themselves, others, and the world. Lack and Bettencourt (1973), Lack (1978), and Allen and O'Dell (1981) describe two different public library programs established in California.

Definition of Bibliotherapy

Having indicated the key features of bibliotherapy as it is understood in this handbook, we can restate our definition: "Bibliotherapy uses literature to bring about a therapeutic interaction between the participant and facilitator." This definition can be expanded as follows: "In interactive bibliotherapy, a trained facilitator uses guided discussions to help the clinical or developmental participant(s) integrate both feelings and cognitive responses to a selected work of literature, which may be a printed text, some form of audiovisual material, or creative writing by the participant."

The discussion thus far should make it clear that there are several assumptions implicit in these definitions:

1. Bibliotherapy is an interactive process.
2. Literature is defined in the broadest sense.
3. The process described takes place in both clinical and developmental bibliotherapy.
4. The practice of bibliotherapy may take place either on a one-on-one basis or in a group setting.
5. The results of effective bibliotherapy are improved self-esteem and assimilation of appropriate psychological or social values into the participant's character and behavior.
6. Bibliotherapy is a *therapy*, but part of its unique effectiveness lies in its use of literature as the primary tool; in this way, bibliotherapy makes a special appeal to the *healthy* aspects of the mind, for both

developmental and clinical participants. As we shall see in the discussion of goals (Chapter 2), the emphasis in interactive bibliotherapy is directed more to the encouragement and reinforcement of strengths than to the diagnosis of problem areas.

7. The effectiveness of bibliotherapy depends on the facilitator's ability to choose material that speaks to the individual participant's needs and interests; to make accurate, empathic interpretations of the participant's responses; and, through literature and dialogue, to draw out deeper self-understanding. In short, a good bibliotherapist is a skilled listener.

Listening in Bibliotherapy

We shall now address in detail the issues raised by this last assumption. During the bibliotherapeutic dialogue, the facilitator must discern not only what the participants *say*—about the literature, about their response, or about the feelings that emerge through discussion—but also what they *mean*. Tone of voice, bearing, nonverbal indicators, and even omissions all reflect what the inner self is feeling and thinking.

Real skill is involved in accurate listening. In the absence of such skill, we often miss the full significance of what another person is saying because we are not at all aware of how our hearing might be blocked by a personal opinion or by an unconscious emotional response to what is being expressed.

Many persons training to do bibliotherapy will have some background in exercising listening skills. Nonetheless, an intellectual understanding of what a given skill calls for is not the same as mastery of that skill. All trainees should expect to learn and to *practice* the kinds of factual and therapeutic listening fundamental to bibliotherapy before conducting any groups. We should note that each discipline in the mental-health field tends to stress certain factors to listen for so that even those with previous training in therapeutic listening can work on becoming sensitive to the particular kinds of messages typical of bibliotherapeutic dialogue.

Six exercises for progressively developing listening skills are given in Appendix A. The primary objective of the first three is to concentrate on what is actually said (facts or content). Basically, each of the three involves listening to an item and reporting on the content with as little personal involvement as possible, so that objectivity dominates. The items called for are three types of material used in bibliotherapy—a factual story, a short story, and a poem.

Only rarely will a facilitator have to report the *content* of the bibliotherapeutic material in this way. However, the facilitator must be able to accurately hear what is said in the dialogue and to accurately communicate the participant's message back to him or her. For the purposes of the exercises, we have found it easier to check accuracy when there is a written text to refer back to. At the same time, a text is more neutral than a verbal exchange between reporter and listener would be, and thus use of a text makes it easier to achieve objectivity.

The second set of three exercises utilizes tapes of the first three sessions. As bibliotherapist, you must not only continue to be aware of objective content but you must also begin to develop the skill of hearing both spoken and unspoken implications, feelings, and nuances. This kind of accurate listening calls for attention to the following points:

- *Tone:* How is the message conveyed?
- *Genre:* What form (i.e., poetry, nonfiction prose, fiction) is chosen, and how does it influence the response?
- *Body Language:* What nonverbal communications accompany the verbal ones? (In other words, is body language relaxed? Rigid? Restless?)
- *Evasiveness:* What is not being said?

The more subtle forms of communication suggested by these four points can be "heard" only with practice. For example, although you might not find it difficult to notice such extremes as a tone of loud anger, attention and experience would be required to pick up quiet anger, particularly in someone who masks his or her emotions. The task is even more demanding when you are trying to decide whether the anger comes from impatience with what is seen as foolishness, from indignation, from a sense of personal grievance, or from self-disgust. Proper identification of the kind of anger involved will depend on your sensitivity as a listener to other elements such as body language, appropriateness of the response to the material, and, of course, the speaker's personality. In short, these messages can be heard only if the objective content of the message is accurately identified.

In addition, the last three exercises are designed to develop an awareness of how easy it is to slip into interpreting material (even when you try not to) instead of reporting objectively. They also call attention to the speaker's capacity to communicate genuine respect and empathy.

Finally, all six exercises are meant to help the bibliotherapist become sensitive to how different genres of literature use different means to communicate different messages. For example, the process of analyzing and reporting what an article is about is quite different from that used in the case of a poem.

Note, too, that the listening exercises use the *tool* of bibliotherapy but do not use it in a bibliotherapeutic way. Specifically, the person who is doing the reporting does not give a *reaction* to the literature—the report is on the *content* of the literature and the purpose is not to be therapeutic but to gauge how well a skill has been mastered. Or, more accurately, it is the *rudimentary basics* of the skill that are being gauged: The ability to listen accurately depends on extensive experience and practice.

All six exercises call for a listening partner. This partner is important in several respects. First, you cannot practice listening unless there is someone to listen to. Second, you are likely to be more observant about specific details when you have to comment on them directly to another person. And, finally, if you find that you resist or resent dealing with the kind of critiquing involved in the exercises, it would be wise to reevaluate your intention to undertake a program that requires outside supervision.

Of course, it is essential that each partner feels confident that the other's observations will be perceptive and honest, and that they will be communicated in a way that is neither abrasive nor destructively negative. If there is a question about a partner's suitability, the issue should be discussed thoroughly and honestly. In some cases, it may be necessary that you make a change.

As valuable as it is to have another's critique, anyone skilled in therapeutic listening must also be capable of self-evaluation. From the beginning, listen to your own responses on the tapes of the listening exercises. Attend both to what has been achieved and to what aspects still need work. Videotapes should be used whenever possible, as they reveal nonverbal behaviors as well as the tone and timbre of the voice. Unless they are being kept to record an individual's progress, training videos can be erased and used many times over.

In addition, as bibliotherapist-in-training you should develop the habit of checking on other listening relationships, such as those with family and friends. It is important that you become aware of how personal feelings can get in the way of accurate listening in ordinary as well as in therapeutic interchanges. Indeed, you need to recognize the personal prejudices you have *against* persons, attitudes, and behaviors as well as those *in favor of* your own concepts and values. As you become conscious of these factors, you can begin to minimize their interference and, hence, maximize your ability to hear accurately.

STUDY GUIDE

1. Discuss how interactive bibliotherapy differs from reading bibliotherapy. Include a definition of therapy.

2. List the main populations that can benefit from interactive bibliotherapy. Then look up and report on one of the in-text sources in which the use of bibliotherapy is described in relation to a population you might be interested in working with.

3. Read and report on one of the following articles, in which the authors provide a basic understanding of bibliotherapy or poetry therapy; then summarize the main points and indicate what you found most useful: Esler (1982), Jalongo (1983b), Morrison (1973), Nickerson (1975), Pattison (1973), Pietropinto (1975), Rubin (1979), Rothenberg (1970, 1972a, 1972b), Sargent (1979), and Silverman (1973, 1977).

PRACTICUM

1. Assume you have heard of a grant for a bibliotherapy project you might carry out. Write a prospectus for this project in which you specify: (a) the population; (b) the setting; (c) the local community forces needed for cooperation; (d) the objectives for the initial series of sessions; and (e) a timetable. Create the kind of project you might actually work on as a volunteer.

2. Using a videotape or a television discussion show as a basis, evaluate in a written report how accurately a selected participant responded to the content of the other members' messages, how able he or she was in hearing more than surface meanings, and what kind of nonverbal messages were used to communicate. In a class situation, ask everyone to report on the same show so that observations can be compared.

FURTHER READINGS

Shiryon (1977a, 1977b) offers another perspective on definition in his discussion of "literatherapy," which he has practiced for twenty-five years. The following oft-cited items in the literature on bibliotherapy consider procedures and effectiveness without distinguishing clearly between reading bibliotherapy and interactive bibliotherapy: Schneck (1945, 1950); Beatty (1962); Favazza (1966); Riggs (1971); Zaccaria and Moses (1978); Sclabassi (1973); Moody (1964); Moody and Limper (1971); Brown (1975); Warner (1980); Schrank and Engels (1981); and Stephens (1981). In addition to the newsletter published by the Bibliotherapy Forum of the American Library Association (see Appendix C), consult journals such as *The Arts in Psychotherapy* for recent developments in bibliotherapy. Banville (1978), Langs (1978), Long (1978), and Shave (1974) are book-length treatments of therapeutic listening skills. The SASHA tapes and Fromm-Reichmann (1950) are also excellent resourses.

We cannot hope to list all the works on concepts of personality and on theories of helping that bibliotherapists should be familar with. Some essential insights can be found, however, in the books by Allport (1955),

Carkhuff (1983), Frank (1973, 1978), Maslow (1962, 1971a), and Yalom (1975, 1980, 1983). Combs (1978), Ellis (1969), Fingarette (1963), Hall and Lindzey (1957), and Wolberg (1967) are other important book-length treatments of theories of personality and therapeutic approaches. Marmor (1975), Ricoeur (1974), and Yarrow (1979) are representative of article-length discussions of the same topics.

2

The Goals of Bibliotherapy

A developmental bibliotherapy group is discussing Naomi Long Madgett's poem "Woman With Flower." The poem begins, "I wouldn't coax the plant if I were you," and then gives precise directives: Too much nurturing may do the plant harm; don't dig the soil up constantly; allow the plant to turn itself toward the sunlight; growth can be stunted by "too much prodding" or too much tenderness. The last line of the poem tells us that we must learn to leave alone the things we love.

After the poem is read aloud, the facilitator invites the participants to take a minute to allow the images in this poem to come to life, using their own imaginations and memories. In different ways, all the participants find that their mental images have been stimulated and enriched by the details of their own lives, which come to mind as they respond to the images. Reflecting on what they recognize in the poem has improved their capacity to respond.

As the discussion turns to the advice in the poem, the focus quickly moves from plant care to personal feelings about what nurturing means. The phrase "I wouldn't," with its personal pronoun, engages even those who are not gardeners. One older woman asserts, "Children need firm direction and guidance. That's the way I was raised and that's what I believe." However, as the discussion goes on, she comes to admit that there are still times when she wonders what she might have done with her life if her father had allowed her to continue her schooling. As others bring up their own experiences, the group members find that the discussion has increased self-understanding.

In discussing the pros and cons of the need to "learn to leave alone" the things we love, one woman shares the pain of standing by her son who is struggling with a drug problem. A man says he has been hurt by his own son's hostile reaction to questions about his activities. "I ask because I'm interested," the man says, "but I'm beginning to wonder if my son thinks I'm checking up on him because I don't trust him."

For all these participants, the bibliotherapy session has increased awareness of interpersonal relationships.

As these group members discuss how they have either forced a relationship or felt prodded by someone else close to them, they find that they are seeing their experiences in a different and more accurate light. The insights triggered by the poem and discussion have uniquely personal implications. But all find that their reality orientation has been improved.

The time is almost up, so the bibliotherapist asks the participants to join in reading the poem aloud. When the last line is read, all take a moment to reflect on the personal insights and goals that have been achieved through the poem and the dialogue.

IN THIS BRIEF ACCOUNT we have pointed to four main goals that the bibliotherapist works to help the participants achieve:

- to improve the capacity to respond by stimulating and enriching mental images and concepts and by helping the feelings about these images to surface
- to increase self-understanding by helping individuals value their own personhood and become more knowledgeable and more accurate about self-perceptions
- to increase awareness of interpersonal relationships
- to improve reality orientation

Each of these goals needs to be examined in detail. But before doing so, we must make two points about them as a whole: The goals are comprehensive, and they are complementary rather than sequential.

As we look at each of the four primary goals of bibliotherapy in turn, we will see that each works with certain needs and areas of the human personality. Yet all four serve one comprehensive purpose—to improve the participants' self-esteem and morale. In other words, bibliotherapy—whether clinical or developmental—shares the overall growth directive common to most therapies. The primary concern is to help the individuals

- have a kindly regard for themselves
- find ways to develop themselves more gracefully
- deal more creatively with what cannot be changed (cf. Frank 1973, 233)

We cannot stress enough the importance of this comprehensive goal. Unfortunately, many normal persons fail to fully recognize and utilize their own strengths even when life is going fairly smoothly. For mentally ill persons, this failure is almost universal.

Low self-esteem becomes an even more serious problem when an individual is faced with conditions that seem unusually difficult. Everyone has a different threshold—circumstances that seem bearable to one will appear to be devastating to another. But, whatever the cause, a state of crisis can trigger feelings of impotence, isolation, despair, and inadequacy. These negative reactions reduce the likelihood that the individual will be able to use any resources he or she does have to act competently. The feeling of being trapped causes further frustration and loss of self-esteem.

Interactive bibliotherapy, with its appeal to the healthy aspects of the personality, can be a factor in breaking this vicious cycle. Ideally, the participant will emerge from a session with a better understanding of the troublesome situation. But even if the problem area has not been dealt with directly, the individual may have responded meaningfully to the material and thus—in this instance, at least—may have successfully engaged in an activity. Every positive experience of coping strengthens morale and self-esteem.

Building the self-esteem of mentally ill people will not, by itself, change their basic defenses, symptoms, or destructive forces of behavior. Nonetheless, if such individuals become more comfortable with themselves, they may be able to respond more successfully to other modes of therapeutic help. Improved self-esteem can help developmental as well as clinical participants improve their capacity to understand and to deal with problems within and outside the context of the bibliotherapy meeting.

Unlike the four steps in the bibliotherapeutic process (to be discussed in the next chapter), the four primary goals of bibliotherapy are complementary rather than sequential; that is, no one goal has inherent priority over the others, nor is there any specified order in which a participant moves from one to the others. Moreover, although an overlap between them often occurs, each of the four goals can be achieved independently.

Furthermore, each of the goals is inexhaustible. No one ever reaches a point where nothing more is to be learned about one's self or one's relationships with others. Our capacity to respond can always be enriched, just as our perceptions of the multiple aspects of reality can always be improved. As we look at each of the major goals of bibliotherapy in turn, it should become even clearer that there are many levels on which each one can be met.

Improving the Capacity to Respond

Improving the capacity to respond is a wide-ranging goal that involves stimulating and enriching the participant's images, concepts, and/or feeling-responses to the bibliotherapeutic materials and to life in general.

In some ways, the first goal is the starting point for the other three: Self-perception, awareness of others, and reality orientation all depend on an initial capacity to respond to the literature and the dialogue. Yet, paradoxically, the end point to which the bibliotherapeutic process tries to bring the participant can also be measured in terms of this goal: If the session has been effective, the participant will be able to respond more fully to his or her insights about self, about relationships with others, or about the reality of his or her life and will be able to demonstrate increased responsiveness by integrating what has been learned.

Because so much is involved in increasing the capacity to respond, we will discuss four aspects of the ways in which this goal is met: Bibliotherapy stimulates the mind and the imagination, allows an experience of the liberating quality of beauty, provides focus, and facilitates the recognition and understanding of feelings.

Mental and imaginative stimulation

Whenever morale is low, the range of interests outside the worry cycle tends to narrow. The literature used in bibliotherapy offers a way of breaking down such self-preoccupation by stimulating both thoughts and imagination. Bibliotherapy participants are engaged by something outside of themselves when they attend to the poem, song, or story that is being presented.

On a very basic level, that "something" can be very tangible. For example, the discussion of a poem about wind made a group of chronic patients aware of the sycamore tree outside the window. On another day, when the weather was dark and stormy, the bibliotherapist directed the dialogue to the patients' response to the sudden gloom. In this way, they came to see that their dislike of the unnatural daytime darkness was perfectly normal. They also discovered that they could decrease their discomfort simply by turning on the lights. The experience became a lesson in the fact that one *can* respond to simple negatives rather than suffer the nameless anxiety that perpetuates dependency.

At other times it is possible, through bibliotherapeutic materials, to introduce a totally new topic or idea—one completely unrelated to the preoccupations of an ill person or the mundane matters of everyday life. Thus a young man struggling with severe depression found release in a discussion of memories brought on by a poem about baseball. As he mentally relived the tremendous excitement he had felt while watching a championship game, he experienced at least temporary release from the lethargy that was overwhelming him.

Or it may be that the fresh input of the literature gives a new perspective to an issue that dominates one's thoughts. For example, in the session reported at the beginning of this chapter, the advice to learn to leave alone what we love was put in terms of caring for a plant; but members of the group found that the recommendation triggered an understanding of their own family relationships.

In all cases, the fresh input encourages healthy use of the imagination. As James Miller has noted:

> To liberate ourselves from *this* moment in time and the immediate range of vision in *this* place, we must use imagination. . . . Without the imagination we would be imprisoned in time and space. . . . With imagination we are enabled, through language, to free ourselves for explorations and discoveries that give meaning to ourselves and our society. (Miller 1972, 5)

In the case of both clinical and developmental groups, then, the introduction of fresh material can provide therapeutic stimulation of thoughts and feelings as the participants are brought to a renewed awareness of the world outside of themselves.

Experiencing the liberating quality of beauty

Frequently, at the same time that the bibliotherapeutic process stimulates the imagination, it enhances the capacity to respond by helping the participants experience the liberating quality of beauty. (We should make it clear, however, that such an experience is not an essential part of every therapeutic interaction in bibliotherapy.) Where beauty is perceived, an integration of self takes place. The integrated personality, by definition, has achieved an ability to *be*—free from the need to possess, to want, to demand for self alone. The same kind of freedom characterizes the recognition of beauty and makes it an integrating experience. By responding to the beauty of a finely crafted poem, story, or play, appreciating the combined sensory and intellectual impact of a film or piece of music, or reflecting on an image that reveals the small beauties of the everyday world, the participant experiences a spontaneous pleasure. As George Santayana (1961, 21–45) has noted, the individual is freed at least momentarily from bondage to the self. And so the soul is glad.

It may seem a simple thing to foster the capacity to enjoy life, to be spontaneous and uninhibited enough to delight in the wonder of a snowflake, the taste of a cold plum, the warmth of a room after the bracing cold of the outdoors. But for many, such simple healthy responses are too rare. At times, the bibliotherapist will feel that facilitating this kind of fundamental response is a sufficient goal for a given session or group. However, the liberating act of experiencing beauty may also release concepts or personal feelings about the topics under discussion. So it is, too, that recognition of the simple delights of the world around us can sharpen our awareness of the deeper wonders of trust, friendship, love, and appreciation.

Providing focus

Bibliotherapy also increases the capacity to respond by providing a focus for attention and aiding in the development of concentration and mental discipline. The capacity to focus varies from individual to individual. People suffering from anxiety and mentally ill individuals often find concentration difficult. Some children may also need help in understanding the advantages of concentrating on one thing at a time in order to learn. Others habitually shy away from looking too deeply within themselves. The bibliotherapist may have to work actively at keeping the discussion focused when dealing with participants who have such difficulties. Other groups will need many fewer interventions to follow through on a subject.

But in all cases, bibliotherapeutic discussion has a focus that is "out there"; in other words, to some extent participants must go outside of themselves to react to an externalized expression of an image, a tale, an emotion, a value. This kind of focused response entails a different level of involvement than the expression of an established preoccupation or of a random and undisciplined flow of thought.

Sustaining focus on a single train of thought often helps the participants clarify their reactions. The act of probing more and more deeply into precisely the personal meaning connected with an idea or feeling not only increases the capacity to respond to the given issue but also provides an experience of what it means to respond on a more intense level.

Recognition and understanding of feelings

Perhaps the most significant way in which bibliotherapy improves the capacity to respond is by helping the participants recognize and understand their feelings. We have already indicated the therapeutic importance of the *feeling-response*. In bibliotherapy, such a response is a dual goal—effective bibliotherapy not only works at the *start* by eliciting a feeling-response but also *results* in a session in which that response has been examined and clarified.

Moreover, there is virtually no limit to the degree of response that can be achieved in terms of this goal. On a very fundamental level, the ability to voice a genuine feeling even about simple things indicates at least a minimal amount of self-confidence. At the same time, acknowledgment of everyday pleasures and fears usually involves some recognition that having these feelings is legitimate rather than a sign of weakness or frivolity.

The expression of *ordinary feelings* will be an achievement for some bibliotherapy participants. We have already suggested how important this kind of recognition can be for clinical patients who either have been institutionalized for a long time or are very withdrawn. But there are many developmental participants, as well, who have been too concerned with practical matters, too preoccupied with worries, or too accustomed to repressing feelings because of what they believe is polite or proper to freely pay attention and express their responses to everyday objects and activities. For such people, the healthy, genuine expression of simple likes and dislikes, pleasures and discomforts, can become the first step in attending to a previously unacknowledged—but very important—aspect of their lives and feelings.

For example, a discussion of Laura Gilpin's poem "Spring Cleaning" may start with the recognition by participants that they, too, save old letters and clothes or with their remembrance of spring cleaning rituals from their pasts. But as the discussion goes on, feelings will emerge. In one case, a patient was able to say that the line about the widow hurt her because she remembered how difficult it had been to give away her husband's things after his death; this woman could begin to free herself some from the pain by expressing something she had not previously felt free to voice. Alcoholics, too, may come to acknowledge that they—like the speaker in the poem—have to "bury those old bones," thus coming to terms with the fact that they have used past hurts to excuse them from acting responsibly in the present.

In addition to ordinary feelings, bibliotherapy can aid participants in the tricky task of acknowledging and dealing with *negative feelings.* Both clinical and developmental participants face situations in which they are unable to act. They may feel helpless or unworthy because of some perceived defect, or they may be paralyzed by ineffectual rage over a harsh reality. One person might conclude that it is hopeless to change what seems so disastrous; another may feel too depressed to hear any positive suggestions about how to improve matters.

Supportive drawing out of negative feelings in a bibliotherapy session allows a participant to express honestly what he or she perceives as reality. The dialogue should help the individual proceed through examination, juxtaposition, and self-application to reassess the negative viewpoint and, ideally, to free him- or herself somewhat from its strictures. It is likely that this process will be long and slow, particularly when the negative feeling is long-standing and/or central to that individual's self-perception.

In many cases, the participant will learn that although the reality cannot be changed, his or her attitude toward it can be. But this solution is not easily come by. Bibliotherapists will have to be clear in their own minds about the almost paradoxical distinction that must be made in response to a negative reality such as loss, illness, or an act of injustice or cruelty. On the one hand, it is both legitimate and basically healthy both to feel and to acknowledge responses such as anger, remorse, hurt, sorrow, and even betrayal. However, it is fundamentally self-destructive to hold on to such feelings in a way that cripples one's ability to cope with and adjust to the reality that caused the emotion. The specific way in which these feelings interact, or the degree to which any one of them is emphasized, will vary from group to group, from session to session, and, above all, from individual to individual.

Increasing Self-Understanding

The second major goal of bibliotherapy is to help participants value themselves and become more accurate about self-perceptions. Erich Fromm (1956) indicates how critical this goal is when he notes that love of self depends on respect, concern, responsibility, and knowledge of self; in addition, he says, there must be a love of self before there is love of others.

Several features of bibliotherapy are particularly suited to meeting this basic therapeutic goal. In the first place, the bibliotherapeutic material offers a unique mirror in which to reflect the participant's self. Second, the dialogue engages the individual in some kind of interaction with this reflection. Clearly, getting in touch with the inner self will not always be a pleasant experience. Sadness and pain are frequently part of the growth process. The familiar discomfort of an unhealthy coping pattern may seem preferable to risking a change; fear will make some participants reluctant to face the challenging experience of dealing with a harsh reality; they may even draw back. Thus, at times, the growth process may seem to result in a retrogression before the next healthy move can be made.

Note that it is through the dialogue in bibliotherapy that the participant signals either retrogression or movement toward deeper understanding. In this therapy, the individual is involved not just with seeing his or her inner self but also with affirming that self by sharing perceptions.

Self-affirmation by simple response

The capacity to make a simple, normal response can be an important achievement for some. Learning-disabled and retarded participants justifiably take pride in their ability to give a simple, coherent response to bibliotherapy material. In general, developmental groups include members who are so painfully shy or afraid of sounding stupid or foolish that they are reluctant to speak up in group situations. But in bibliotherapy, previously held inhibitions are often freed: First, the affirmative climate that characterizes each bibliotherapy session makes it easier to talk. Second, the discussion begins more neutrally when the participants are asked for a feeling-response to the literature than when group members are told to bring up a problem or are quizzed about content.

But even a simple response can be an especially meaningful expression of self-affirmation in clinical settings. Just as muscles atrophy without use, the capacity to respond normally can be crippled by life in an institution, where few opportunities exist for normal, personal decisions and responses related to everyday matters. Scheduled bibliotherapy sessions in which basic, reality-oriented responses are expected and achieved create such an opportunity.

Over time, even very withdrawn patients will begin to offer some kind of "normal" response to the literature and the dialogue. For example, in a group of blind, mentally ill patients, one man was passed an object meant to make the day's material more vivid. Initially he recognized the jingle bells on a leather strap through sound and feeling and said he remembered seeing such straps when he was young, when there were horses in Baltimore—"but not for years," he added. He then sang several verses of "Jingle Bells" while a couple of the other patients, ordinarily very silent, joined in. For both the man and the singers, this much of a response was a significant achievement. And as the pleasure on their faces indicated, it was one that made them feel better. The therapeutic benefit was not that they were dealing with a problem area but that they were freed, at least briefly, to experience a simple, healthy delight.

Self-affirmation through recollection of the past

In the example just given, the therapeutic response grew out of a memory. In fact, bibliotherapy often involves some kind of helpful working out of memories. The stimulus to remember may come from something in the literature, or it may be the result of a creative writing assignment specifically designed to elicit memories.

The simple recollection of the past is particularly meaningful for certain populations. Developmental groups of senior citizens also often find strength in memories (Merriam 1980; Lewis and Butler 1974). So, too, the experience of voicing memories often gives institutionalized patients a distinct sense of each others' identities for the first time—and this is the case even when group members have lived together for years on the same hospital ward. As one person talks of picking strawberries and packing them for sale and another remembers babies in the field as the mothers picked cotton along the row, or as yet a third man talks of his tailoring business and another remembers what it was like before his law business failed, all the group members become aware of themselves as having a unique store of memories of the everyday details of their lives.

The process of going over memories in the context of a bibliotherapy discussion is therapeutic in many ways. On one level, the focusing brought about by the therapeutic process itself can make memories rewarding. In addition, the material gives a certain structure and frame of reference to the discussion so that the memories are not haphazard. Finally, as the facilitator guides the exchange, there is some sense of purpose in the session.

Participants' responses will vary as well. Some participants may find new strength in reliving a meaningful past moment; others may discover that a long-forgotten experience can help them appreciate more fully some aspect of their present lives. In some cases, the acknowledgment of a difficult past moment might even become the first step toward dealing with an unresolved issue or establishing new patterns. Alternatively, the participant may find strength and affirmation in the discovery that an experience or quality that had been a source of distress in the past no longer has power over the present self. In still other cases, a participant will be comforted by discovering that others find his or her response to the memory to be legitimate. For example, comforting (and often silent) approval is frequently given in bibliotherapy sessions in response to the weeping of a participant—which in itself is usually a healthy response to sorrow.

Self-affirmation through opinion-giving

Expressing an opinion is usually the most direct way in which participants discover and assert their inner selves. Feeling free enough to give a personal opinion requires not only the reporting of a directly verifiable "what happened" but also the assertion of one's understanding of the more nebulous "how" and "why." For example, a discussion of Carl Sandburg's poem "Soup" might begin with observations that work out of such questions as: Where was the man when he ate his soup? Or, did he eat it alone or with others? However, in declaring, "That man isn't that different from me," or even "I don't like eating soup," a participant takes the risk of evaluating and asserting something that can be verified only by reference to his or her own feelings.

Bibliotherapy seems to offer a particularly safe environment for developing the capacity to express opinions. In the first place, the emphasis is on opinion and feeling rather than on objective verification of content. Furthermore, participants do not have to begin by directly confronting one another. At first, one can say, "I don't agree with the writer." Then, "My reaction is different from yours." Exchanging responses about a poem may help individuals clarify for themselves as well as for others what they were trying to express.

Often, opinions are not only expressed but examined as well. In the process of saying with increasing accuracy, "This is what I feel; this is what I believe," the individual comes closer to both defining and affirming the self.

As alcohol- and chemical-dependency programs emphasize, expressing opinions is most therapeutic when the participant is willing to personalize the statement. The bibliotherapist may have to work hard to get participants to see why "Speaking for myself, I see this as. . . ." is a better response than "People say that. . . ." The personalized opening in the first example indicates that the speaker is willing to take responsibility for—and be identified with—the opinion being voiced.

Clarifying Personal Relationships

Human beings are social animals—in John Donne's words, "No man is an Island." And, we can add, no man will understand himself if he does not understand himself as one person in a world peopled with others. A sense of identity requires another by whom one is known. Bibliotherapy furthers this third goal—improvement of the participant's awareness of interrelationships—in a process consisting of three stages.

Developing awareness of feelings as universal

Anxiety is often accompanied by the sense that the individual is the only one who has ever had to deal with the emotion, problem, or situation that is so troubling. But as participants listen to the material presented in a bibliotherapy session and join in the dialogue, some kind of recognition usually takes place. Perhaps a character in the story or film seems to be facing the same kind of troubles they are experiencing; maybe a phrase or image seems to echo a reaction they have had, or the feelings described are their feelings. In any case, the individual participant discovers a shared reference point. Another person, the one who wrote or composed what has just been read or heard, has conveyed something identifiable to the participant. Even if the feeling or situation is not resolved in a way that applies directly to the individual, knowing that the experience has been shared by others eases the sense of isolation.

In time, if the bibliotherapeutic experience is positive and supportive, a withdrawn participant may also become aware of the facilitator, who in turn responds empathically, and accurately, to what the person is saying. The facilitator is both more immediate and more personally responsive than an impersonal author. As the participants learn to use the facilitator's help in expressing and dealing with their problems, they are simultaneously learning that the feelings being shared are not so crippling as they may have seemed. To adapt Buber's eloquent phrase, the bibliotherapeutic dialogue brings about "healing through meeting" (Buber 1963; Friedman 1976).

Note that the bibliotherapist need not always share the exact feelings that were expressed. Sometimes the response will be: "That is a different way of looking at things. I had not thought of that. Tell us more." This reaction affirms that it is both possible and legitimate to have unique reactions; yet it also suggests that such reactions need not isolate the speaker—he or she can be heard by another.

Developing awareness of others

The recognition that one can be *heard* is the most elementary stage in developing awareness of others. The awareness increases significantly at the point where the participant sees that *listening* is also possible. Although it is a sign of serious mental illness to be completely withdrawn from the world outside of oneself, it is by no means unusual to find individuals who have little awareness of how they are seen by others and even less sensitivity to how others are affected by them.

For very ill persons or for children, adolescents, or others caught up in narcissism, the bibliotherapist may begin by setting the goal of working on the *basic socialization skills* that make group discussion possible. Thus participants might be asked to help set up the seating arrangement for the group and to share copies of the literature and the pictures or tactile objects that are being used to heighten the effect of the selection. It may be necessary to spell out ground rules such as these: Participants may not interrupt a speaker either by speaking or by behaving in a distracting manner; no one may leave the group before the session is over. Enforcing the rules in a firm and respectful way may seem to aim at little more than behavior modification. But the message that the bibliotherapist will articulate sometimes and leave implicit at other times is that the underlying rationale for the rules is not merely logistical: We acknowledge and respect others because everyone has value; furthermore, we can learn something for ourselves by attending to others because we all share certain experiences and feelings.

Even in groups in which basic ground rules are easily established, it may still be necessary to work on facilitating true group interactions. If members tend to direct their responses only to the leader, the bibliotherapist will refer questions and responses back to other group members whenever possible. Again, the emphasis is on strengthening the individual's awareness of others as also having feelings and responses.

In both developmental and clinical groups, some participants are reluctant to speak because of their fear of others' reactions. The fear can stem from wanting to avoid the shame of saying something "wrong," or it may come from the feeling that disagreement necessarily means disapproval. Here the bibliotherapist must work to establish the assumptions that govern a therapeutic climate for discussion—namely, that participants recognize that there are no "right" or "wrong" answers but only genuine ones; that what one says is often recognized as true for someone else; but also that, in any case, there is a value in honest differences. Explaining to another what one means often clarifies one's own convictions; besides, saying "I personally see or feel things differently" is not the same as saying "What you said is of no value."

In other words, as members of a bibliotherapy group listen, consider, and respond both to the literature and to others' remarks, they should experience, at least to some extent, the therapeutic value of acknowledging others. If reactions can be shared, if someone else's response can be valid though different, if another viewpoint can be tolerated, then one is neither hopelessly isolated nor trapped by one's own responses. Equally important, by acknowledging others, we open ourselves to consolation from another.

Developing awareness of feelings for others

To be fully human we cannot just be aware *of* others. We must also feel *for* them. The fact is, one's day-to-day existence is deeply involved with others. The way we feel about interdependence and sharing clearly has an effect on how we live and respond. At the very least, if we try to ignore how we react to and feel about others, we are denying a significant part of our experience, whether positive or negative.

Now, most of us recognize at least intellectually how empty life is without love or compassion. Still it can be difficult to acknowledge how much we all need others. The dialogue that is central to the bibliotherapeutic process, as well as the content of many items used as material, clearly testifies that not all dependency is crippling. Yet it is also essential to good mental health that we acknowledge the existence of people we don't like and the interdependencies we find irritating or stifling. It is equally important that we periodically assess such feelings.

Bibliotherapy can be a useful vehicle for dealing with such issues. A song, a poem, or a story can help us recognize more precisely what it is that we dislike. Then we can determine whether that dissatisfaction is with the self, with something from the past, or with the person or situation at hand.

Both clinical and developmental groups will include participants who are very aware of what they believe to be others' feelings about them. However, self-absorbed persons tend neither to check the reality behind their perceptions nor to recognize the legitimate needs others may have. As such individuals are led by the bibliotherapeutic dialogue to look at relationships in a story or film, they may begin to be aware of the importance of integrating their own needs with those of others.

One particular example concerning a clinical participant comes to mind. Lois was extremely shy and withdrawn; she answered if spoken to directly and was alert in the bibliotherapy sessions but never proffered any personal reactions. Up to this point, moreover, the staff had been unsuccessful in their attempts to get her to recontact her family and to make specific plans to return to her home community in view of her scheduled release after years of hospitalization.

In this particular session, the facilitator read Betty Wilkinson's poem, "Why Do They?" After asking a series of questions about why other people keep to themselves, the poem concludes, "Why do they? Why do I?"

The facilitator worked hard to develop feeling-responses to phrases in the poem about persons looking the other way, wearing masks, and not showing their desires. But the discussion was desultory, and the group members were not really able to verbalize the connection between their own behavior and that of others. Lois herself said little during the discussion. However, as the session ended, she came up close to the facilitator and very intently said, "Why do I?" and then left the group.

The facilitator learned later that immediately following the meeting, Lois had left the hospital grounds, gone to the local bus depot some distance away, and returned to her home in another state. Lois's family called the hospital that evening, delighted to have her return. (Subsequently, Lois did come back to the hospital for a few more weeks of guidance to prepare her for the transition to life as an out-patient in her own community. But, in contrast to her previous behavior, she became actively involved in the programs scheduled for her.)

Although she did not respond aloud in the discussion, Lois seems to have made a sharp application to herself of the question "Why do I?" This line from the poem triggered an insight about her self-absorption and how it had led her to treat others. She was then able to determine for herself that she should change her response to the outside world. Although the entire treatment team had initiated Lois's improvement by preparing her to return to life in the community, it was only when she recognized her personal responsibility to others that she was actually able to act.

This is an unusually dramatic example of how bibliotherapy can help individuals improve personal relationships. Even so, there are many sessions in which the therapist both sets and meets goals that involve helping individuals communicate with others in order to better understand themselves and to gain a clearer picture of their relationship to others.

Enlarging Reality Orientation

There is a temptation to think of the fourth major goal of bibliotherapy as applying primarily to disturbed people. However, all of us can profit at times from correcting our perception of the world around us. Children or adolescents may well have problems in seeing just how they relate to the world of adults. And "normalized" adults find again and again that there are many different ways to look at reality and that it is not always easy to keep the different facets of one's world in perspective. So, too, the normal aging person has been through many phases of personhood and may welcome the opportunity to use the perspective of literature and his or her own insights to analyze the present.

There are a number of levels on which this goal can be met, depending on the nature of the group and of the individual participants. We will now consider each of these levels in turn.

Relating coherently to concrete images or information

As indicated earlier, bibliotherapy can be a very effective means of helping regressed or deeply disturbed persons relate to reality in a very tangible way. Materials such as D. Aldis's poems "Hands" and "Feet" or C. Morley's "Smells" deal with concrete everyday objects. They usually have an immediate impact and stimulate some verbalized response. For patients who are wrapped up in their delusions, focusing on an exterior reality can be a real achievement. Or the activity as a whole may allow a clinical participant to show certain strengths. Some chronic patients, retarded group members, or others who have tended to be dreamy or unresponsive in groups oriented toward problem-solving may remember, say, that the bibliotherapy group meets on Wednesdays in the alcove at 3 P.M.—although this may be one of the few times and places they voluntarily relate to. Once at the meeting, moreover, they may be able to attend to the materials, comment on each other's presence or absence, and in general keep to the subject of the discussion. All of these actions attest to at least a minimal ability to relate to external reality and, as such, are therapeutic.

Relating to social, psychological, and emotional realities

The bibliotherapist hopes to go beyond recognition of such tangible realities. Group members will be urged to use their conscious thoughts and memories as a means to examine the more complex—and potentially more troubling—realities of their emotional, social, and psychological lives. For example, a striking image may prompt us to realize that we must examine whether or not we have truly let go of a feeling that we describe as being in the past. In other cases, a situation in a story under discussion reveals that our expectations for the future are unrealistic. Or the discussion of yet another work may help us see that we have rewritten the past in an attempt to deny a motive that we are ashamed of.

Frequently, a bibliotherapy group opens with a logical explanation offered by a participant as to why something happened or why some attitude or action is "correct." But as the discussion goes on, members come to see that logic alone is not enough to account for the reality of the feeling-response in question. A part of learning to deal with reality involves one's learning to probe facile explanations as to why situations and relationships turn out as they do.

In effect, bibliotherapy focuses on helping participants face what Irvin Yalom (1975) calls the "existential issues." Yalom based his analysis on the issues that his clients reported they felt had to be recognized if they were to cope successfully. These issues include the following:

- Life is at times unfair and unjust.
- Ultimately there is no escape from pain and death.
- No matter how close I get to others, I still must face life alone.
- I must face the issues of my life and death, and therefore live life more honestly and be less embroiled in trivialities.
- I must take the ultimate responsibility for the way I live my life, regardless of the support and guidance I get from others.

The struggle for maturity almost always involves a coming to terms with one or more of these issues. More than that, the mature person is characterized by his or her ability to continually translate these realities into coping patterns. The literature and the dialogue are useful vehicles both for examining the existential issues and for exploring ways in which to integrate them.

In a sense, then, every bibliotherapy session will regard the improvement of reality orientation as one of its goals. It could even be argued that the fourth goal is inseparable from the other three. The more realistically we relate to the world outside of ourselves, the more able we are to respond to that world; as we grow in our understanding of ourselves and of our relationships with others, we are coming to terms with our personal realities.

Using the Goals

When setting general goals for a group and specific goals for a given session or participant, keep these four important points in mind.

Goals are not programmable

Establishing goals for bibliotherapy involves a number of fairly fine distinctions. On the one hand, a good bibliotherapist is aware not just of the four overall goals but also of the kind of precise objectives that we list for each of the four in our discussion of criteria in Chapter 4. Moreover, in planning for a session, the facilitator does have specific goals and objectives in mind both for the group as a whole and for individual members.

For example, the bibliotherapist who planned the developmental session that opened this chapter chose Madgett's poem because she felt it would be an effective tool for helping group members focus on the third main goal by examining the interpersonal issue of dependence/independence—an issue that many of them had indicated was critical for them. She also felt that the concrete images and personal pronouns in the poem would further the objective she had for helping one of the women members begin to personalize her responses, rather than focusing on the structure of the work in literary terms.

Of course, there is an important distinction between setting goals and establishing a preconceived timetable. In other words, the bibliotherapist should not decide to devote the first three sessions of a group to enhancing the capacity to respond and the next three to increasing awareness of self. Such scheduling would undercut the facilitator's responsiveness to the therapeutic possibilities that come from each unique blend of literature and dialogue.

Goals are not quantifiable

In the necessary process of reviewing and evaluating how well the goals have been met, the bibliotherapist must keep a sense of proportion. In the first place, he or she should recognize from the outset that the capacity to measure therapeutic effect is very limited. In a later chapter we do provide charts for measuring the participant's progress, but these instruments look at *patterns* of response rather than attempt any kind of grading. Particularly with clinical groups, it is hard to be sure that any goal was met to any significant extent.

For example, in the case involving Lois, bibliotherapy seems to have been a critical factor in rendering the patient able to return to her community. But note that the effectiveness of the procedure was *not* observable to the bibliotherapist at the time.

By the same token, other individuals may respond well to the literature in the atmosphere of the bibliotherapy group but show little change in general ward behavior or life situations. In one case, a very regressed patient had not participated at all throughout the many months she had been in the group. But she suddenly responded eloquently to a brief description of Maggie L. Walker's successful efforts to organize a bank for blacks in Richmond in 1903. The patient described in detail the difficulties she herself had had years before in another southern city when she had tried to bank her wages. From that point on, the same woman made relevant comments when the topic interested her. However, it took a year and a half for this patient to modify even slightly her withdrawn and hostile behavior on the ward.

Goals are inexhaustible

But aside from how difficult it is to measure therapeutic success, there are many facets to each goal and each facet operates on many levels. Thus, although it is possible to note progress in one direction or another, the facilitator can never assume that an individual has "finished with" any one of the goals.

The fact that the goals are inexhaustible is closely linked to the overall growth directive to which they all contribute. The task of becoming more fully, more competently, more comfortably ourselves never can be finished because life is not static. Then again, bibliotherapy is effective precisely because of the flexible nature of its main tool—the literature that is the starting point for dialogue is always open to a new reading.

Goals are therapeutic, not diagnostic

Finally, we must reiterate an important point about the goals of bibliotherapy as presented in this handbook: We do not deal with the ways in which bibliotherapy might be used as a tool to help the facilitator assign a specific label, such as those found for psychiatrists in the *Diagnostic and Statistical Manual of Mental Disorders.* Rather, we confine ourselves to the therapeutic goals of drawing out and reinforcing the individual's strengths to resolve the problem areas that have emerged.

STUDY GUIDE

1. List the overall growth directives for bibliotherapy. Then read Frank (1974) and analyze the reasons for which the overall growth directives are valuable for both clinical and developmental participants.
2. Briefly state your understanding of the use of bibliotherapy to increase the capacity to respond.
3. State your understanding of the use of bibliotherapy to enlighten either personal relationships or the process of self-affirmation.
4. Indicate the relationship you see between Yalom's existential issues (listed in the section entitled "Relating to social, psychological, and emotional realities") and bibliotherapy.

PRACTICUM

1. Analyze Miller's (1972) statement on imagination in the section entitled "Mental and Imaginative Stimulation." Use examples of bibliotherapeutic materials to apply the statement specifically to what will happen in bibliotherapy sessions. Be prepared to consult some of the works on the function of imagery and the imagination given in "Further Readings."
2. Read Crootof (1969) to visualize a bibliotherapy session. Choose a bibliotherapy item. Review how you might see the four goals emerge in a session, using the example at the beginning of the chapter as a general model. Be sure to refer to your chosen item to demonstrate different points.

FURTHER READINGS

For literary theory on the function of imagery and imagination, read articles from Kosinski (1968), Rugg (1963), Gallagher (1980), and Ricoeur (1978). Singer (1971, 1973, 1975a) provides a valuable review of how "imagery" has been used in psychiatry. Other psychologically oriented discussions include Rogers (1973), Jung (1968), McKellar (1957), Shorr (1980), and Strawson (1970). Silverman (1977) discusses the relationship between imagery and the bibliotherapeutic goals and process; Van Tichelt (1977) concludes that imagery "as a variable may have great bearing on the effects of bibliotherapy." Jaskoski (1980) discusses the reasons for which a poetry therapist should be trained in analysis and interpretation of poetry as well as in therapeutic skills. Branden (1969) offers a book-length treatment of the concept of self-esteem. Finally, Plutchik (1980) and Plessner (1970) deal with the processes involved in expressing feelings, whereas De Rosis (1978) devotes one chapter to suggesting specific techniques for helping patients work on their feelings.

3

The Bibliotherapeutic Process

As I listen to my developmental group discussing "Devotion" by Robert Frost, I am struck by both the simplicity and the brevity of the poem. In particular, my attention is arrested by the first of the four lines in which the poet establishes a metaphor between devotion and the relationship between the shore and the ocean. I recognize that there is something here that interests me. Others ask questions.

I listen; I both agree with and question what others have said so far. It is time now to examine what personal understanding this poem and the dialogue about it can bring to us.

I say, "Heart can mean both love and hate." Another woman says, "But the word devotion *can only mean one thing—steadfastness."*

We go on to examine other paradoxes in the poem and in ourselves. I find myself juxtaposing *my feelings and my analysis of both feelings and ideas with the ideas and reactions expressed by other members of the group.*

As the discussion continues, I begin to see how I agree and disagree with things that have been said. The others are doing the same and coming to some understanding of what is true for them personally. We are all engaged in a process of self-application.

I say what I suddenly realize I feel strongly. "I know what endless repetition *means to me in this poem. It is like the beat of the heart. THUMP, THUMP, THUMP—steady and measured the way the heart has to beat for us to stay alive. That's the way I want my love to be—like waves pounding against the immovable shoreline."*

A young man slowly says, "I still don't feel that. . . ."

The facilitator says, "Our time is up now. But in the coming days, each of you might think about what you learned about yourself from this discussion. We'll continue this theme next week with another poem."

THE STEPS IN THE BIBLIOTHERAPEUTIC PROCESS are fourfold: After a participant's attention is caught by something in the reading (recognition), he or she goes on to look at the issues and the personal feeling-response to them (examination). The process then moves to a deeper level of understanding as the person considers the first level of understanding in light of any new feelings or ideas that emerge in the dialogue (juxtaposition). Finally the individual evaluates the impressions and insights and integrates them into his or her inner self (self-application). The whole process culminates in a new, deeply personal meaning that will inform future attitudes and actions.

It is as Robert Frost says in the foreword to his *Selected Poems:* "A poem begins in delight and ends in wisdom."

The Bibliotherapeutic Process Versus Education and Therapy

The kind of wisdom that comes from bibliotherapy specifically addresses an understanding of the self rather than a grasp of the nature of the world at large. By the same token, the process through which understanding emerges must not be confused with what takes place either in a classroom discussion of literature or in a traditional therapy session.

In a class, the interaction takes place between the student-literature-teacher; the literature is usually considered to be the *object* of discussion rather than a *tool.* The teacher's goal is to help the student achieve some insight into the meaning and value of the work as written. Discussion might focus on historical context, nature of the genre, structure, use of imagery or language, or presentation of dominant themes.

In bibliotherapy, however, the value of the literature depends strictly on its capacity to encourage a therapeutic response from the participants. The individual's feeling-response is more important than an intellectual grasp of the work's meaning. Thus, in bibliotherapy even a misinterpretation of the text will be considered both legitimate and useful if it leads to the release of feelings or insights related to self-understanding. In other words, the use of literature in bibliotherapy reflects the goals of therapy rather than those of education.

But there is an equally important distinction between bibliotherapy and classical modes of therapy. In most therapies, either the therapist or the client raises a psychological issue and focuses directly on it in a way that makes the client acknowledge and, ultimately, resolve the problem area. The triad here might be designated as participant-problem-therapist. There is no intermediary tool in this context, as there is in bibliotherapy.

Literature as a Catalyst in the Bibliotherapeutic Process

In effect, the literature is a *catalyst*; that is, the text, in and of itself, is neither therapeutic nor altered by the process of bibliotherapy. The therapeutic effect depends on the *response to* the literature as it is facilitated through the dialogue, and the change takes place in the *respondent*.

As we examine each step in the bibliotherapeutic process, we will see that such a catalyst has particular advantages for therapeutic dialogue. Specifically, the process is expedited by the fundamentally affirmative, flexible and non-coercive qualities of the literature. In the first place, participants are not directed to see themselves in terms of their problems but, rather, are invited to respond to a poem, story, essay, article, or film. The message implicit in such an invitation is that the participants have competence and worth: They are capable of responding to something outside of themselves, and they can offer accurate and helpful interpretations of the material. In essence, the literature and the dialogue become vehicles for hope, which William Lynch (1965) sees as a matter of "imagining the real."

At the same time, effective literature is rich with all kinds and levels of meaning. The participant is free either to reflect on a problem area or to affirm a strength. While the bibliotherapist works to draw out or deepen both the level of response and the way it is processed, the literature gives the participant some autonomy—as individual reactions cannot be programmed.

Finally, literature naturally seems to invite a deeply *personal response*. Holland (1975), Rosenblatt (1976, 1978), and Shrodes (1949) are among those who see reading as a continuing *process*, not as a passive act. They emphasize somewhat different points, but all three are concerned with exploring how the reader's self, or personality, affects the way in which the literature is absorbed. These studies concentrate explicitly on the act of reading, but our point is that the spontaneous response (which does indeed reflect self) can be deepened and developed *through the dialogue* that characterizes interactive bibliotherapy. In fact, in interactive bibliotherapy the focus is not so much on the initial stimulus as on the *process* of working through the recognition to some kind of integrated understanding.

Note, too, that the concept of process used here is not tied to any specific school or approach. The manner in which the participant interacts with the literature is the same regardless of whether the facilitator interprets the response as Freudian, Jungian, Adlerian, or eclectic.

Step One: Recognition

The bibliotherapeutic process begins with an initial recognition: There is something in the material that *engages* the participant—something that piques interest, opens the imagination, stops wandering thoughts, or in some way arrests attention. At the same time, it is critical in bibliotherapy that the "something" being recognized is the understanding of a person or an experience rather than of the piece of literature as such.

Thus, the participant is not expected to say, "I've heard that poem before" or "I saw that film last year"; rather, the hope is that he or she will declare, "I've felt helpless just like the man in the story," or "There's something in the refrain that really haunts me." As Frost says in a single succinct line: "The initial delight [of a poem] is in the surprise of remembering something I didn't know I knew" (Frost 1963, 3).

Frost's line points to one of the advantages associated with the use of a catalyst. Because responses are unrehearsed and spontaneous, the participant may be *surprised* into a recognition. In some instances, the participant becomes aware of a concept or piece of information for the first time. In other cases, the surprise comes from dealing with something that had seemed too commonplace to consider before. The fact is, our lives are filled with apparently mundane activities. Reflecting on what these details mean to us—what they make us feel and/or remember—can put us in touch with ourselves in an important way.

Sometimes it is just one single aspect of a selection rather than the whole work that strikes a chord. For example, one line of a poem reverberates: "How can we know the dancer from the dance?" Nothing else is remembered, not even the seemingly unrelated title of William Butler Yeats's "Among School Children." In other cases, it will not even be an isolated image or line but simply the rhythm that opens up some kind of understanding.

There is some variation in the way in which the recognition comes. At times, it is immediate. In other cases, the literature itself does not directly spark a catalytic response. The facilitator may have to probe a bit before any recognition takes place. Or the remarks of other members in a group may stir a response. However, even when the response comes through the dialogue, it is still the literature that initiated the discussion and thus can be considered a catalyst.

Whatever the impetus, the specific nature of the recognition can vary enormously. We will consider only three important kinds of recognition that can be initiated by the literature and dialogue.

Unacknowledged feelings

Bibliotherapy is a particularly effective catalyst for helping participants recognize and deal with the ambiguities that normal growth demands—and that many persons never come to terms with precisely because the issues are ambiguous.

For example, "Love in a Plain Wrapper," by Susan McGinnis, depicts a wife aware of her deep love for her husband. But she does not surround herself with romance—her perfume is the steam from the boiling pot. And rather than tell him that she loves him, "Instead, I give you your dinner." There are as many ways to respond to the issues implicit in this poem as there are men and women in the group discussing it. The image of love and happiness in an ordinary domestic setting might be the catalyst that enables one woman to acknowledge the guilt she feels because the poem is *not* true for her, even though she regards the attitudes expressed as an ideal. Another finds an image that helps him formulate feelings about his wife that he had not been able to voice before. In the course of discussion one woman may test how others react to the fact that her feelings about her marriage waver back and forth. Someone else will see the poem as the perfect image of her concept of love through service, whereas still another might find that an examination of the instantaneous negative reaction he had to the poem offers some insight into the ambivalence he actually feels about the way he and his wife have been trying to avoid traditional roles in their marriage.

It is true not only that participants respond in different ways but also that individual reactions are triggered by different lines or themes of the poem; similarly, the degree to which the recognition touches on a critical area varies. But the theme and treatment offer an effective tool for coming to terms with a universal psychological reality—namely, that personal feelings about human relationships and situations are seldom clear-cut.

Recognizing patterns of response

In other cases, the very act of repeatedly engaging in the bibliotherapeutic process triggers recognition of a pattern of response. For example, over the course of several sessions, it may become clear that a particular person habitually complains about the selections or sees only somber messages in the literature. The bibliotherapy group offers a clear context in which to help such an individual recognize that his or her spontaneous response tends to be negative. Particularly in the case of clinical participants, this kind of attitude may be very deep-seated. Although the facilitator should not expect to effect a cure, the literature can serve as a catalyst for some kind of limited change. For example, the individual might agree to try to find at least one positive element in the material used at each session.

Catharsis

At times, the recognition brought about by the literature is so strong as to bring about a catharsis. But before giving examples of such a response, we should first clarify the terminology. *Catharsis* was first used by Aristotle to describe the process by which sympathetic identification with the tragic hero can release emotions and thereby create feelings of purification (catharsis is the Greek word meaning "cleansing"). In psychiatric terms, catharsis refers to the release of thoughts and feelings that have been suppressed;

the surfacing of unconscious materials is accompanied by an emotional response and a release from tension (Simon 1978). The stimulus that brings about this release is not specifically linked to literature, however.

In bibliotherapy, we understand catharsis as having overtones of both a literary and a psychological meaning. The release that is experienced may come from a strong identification with something in the work or from the way the work or the dialogue about it touches a buried memory or emotion. But in either case there is a link between the material used and the strong emotional impact.

As employed here, the term *catharsis* means a profound experience of recognition. The following case involving one member of a group of alcoholics will illustrate both the power and the limitation of this therapeutic response.

The first time Jack attended a bibliotherapy group, in this instance one that was functioning as part of a thirty-five-day alcoholic treatment program, another member had picked a poem called "Loneliness" from Thomas Boyd's collection, *Windows, Walls, Bridges*. As other members dialogued about their previous need to be "people-pleasers" and about their reluctance to be alone, Jack looked on. He seemed aloof as well as somewhat hostile. When addressed, he said he did not see much relevance in the poem to his life.

The next week, the bibliotherapist used another work from the same booklet; this poem began by thanking those "who had understood me," and also, later, those who could not understand. Again, the group members mentioned particular persons in their lives to whom the various lines might be addressed. Jack, however, was quite forceful (albeit pleasant) in saying that he could not see how you could thank anyone who had not understood you. Then he added, rather proudly, "I have never been lonely. I am quite self-sufficient." He went on to describe how he got tired of being around people. More than once he had climbed into his van and taken to the woods to hunt for weeks on end, "Till it gets to me and I feel I can't stand being alone any longer. Then I come out, but I'm not lonely."

Others in the group mentioned that they did miss the family they no longer saw. They were talking quietly, matter of factly. Then quite abruptly Jack exclaimed, "Say, have any of you ever felt this way?" He stopped and then went on more slowly, "I've never asked anyone else this before. But as you're riding along in traffic, has a pang ever struck you? A real pain—it almost takes your breath away. And suddenly, for no reason you know of, you realize this pain comes from missing someone you haven't seen for years."

Almost all of the group members nodded in agreement and began to express their own experiences. For the first time since he joined the group, Jack really listened to the others. He spoke at length of his overdependence on a woman friend who had left him. He said he had not seen that she was unable to cope with such dependency. Slowly he said, as the session closed, "So that is loneliness."

As real as his catharsis had been, Jack left the program shortly after this session. He was not able to move beyond recognition of the loneliness and dependency he had so vehemently denied to an integration that would let him act on his insight.

This case illustrates several important points. In the first place, although the literature can be an important factor in bringing about catharsis, the participant is ultimately responsible for the response. Moreover, catharsis, like other kinds of recognition, is only the first step in an extended process in which the individual must be willing to engage before a change in behavior can occur.

This case is also a striking example of how the literature alone did not bring about recognition; it was clear that the *dialogue about* the literature was the actual catalyst.

Jack's response was cathartic in the sense generally employed in psychiatry. But catharsis in interactive bibliotherapy does not always depend on the surfacing of unconscious material. At times, the recognition comes through a spontaneous emotional response to the beauty or poignancy of a scene or emotion depicted in the literature. In one case, Kenneth Rexroth's translation of a Japanese haiku brought tears of wonder to the eyes of a participant and served as the impetus for a powerful recognition of the concept that life might be so long and difficult that present unhappy times should actually be fondly recalled. This restatement of the message may not seem very striking. But what moved this participant was the poetic expression of the idea: The catharsis seems to have come from the liberating quality of beauty itself.

Time and again, this will happen—a poem, a story, or a film will trigger recognition not so much through its message but because of the power with which the theme or idea is expressed.

Recognition as an individualized process

There is one final point to make about recognition in bibliotherapy: The bibliotherapist looks for literature that is universal enough, beautiful enough, profound but true enough to touch each individual in a group; he or she also facilitates the discussion to make the most of the material's potential. Ultimately, however, recognition cannot be programmed. The human heart is too singular.

Yet it is because the process is by definition personal that the flexibility of the tool becomes a real therapeutic advantage. The recognition can be immediate and deeply significant or it can take place more slowly and on a more concrete level. Thus, some participants must grow to feel safe in making simple observations about concrete, nonthreatening images and ideas before they can give a feeling-response. Others are able to deal with an idea or feeling "out there" because it is expressed in neutral terms through the literature, whereas they would be defensive if the same point were raised directly.

Step Two: Examination

As we casually read, watch films, or listen to songs, there are many details we recognize but deliberately do not examine. It may be that we just want to relax, or that reflection would be too painful or would take too much time and work. However, in bibliotherapy we must move beyond the flash of recognition to *examine* the concept or feeling for ourselves. We must explore what the feeling-response we have recognized actually means to us.

Examination involves the questions who, what, when, why, how, how much, and wherefore. If we examine something as concrete as a stone, we look at its surface; we turn it over and look at the underside; we feel it; we notice its smoothness or roughness, its shape, its weight, its size. Although feelings are more tenuous than the characteristics of a stone, the examination of them is far more necessary—and it is equally necessary to specify the different facets of the initial recognition.

In effect, the second step of the process is an intensification of the first. For example, a participant immediately recognized that he was initially deeply angered by James Thurber's humorous fable "The Courtship of Arthur and Al." He was aware that he was especially put off by the moral, "It is better to have loafed and lost than never to have loafed at all." But as he was led to examine his reaction more closely in the dialogue, the man came to see that *what* really disturbed him was the attitude implicit in the moral—an attitude that had bothered him on several occasions *when* other people in his office were able to joke about a business loss over which he had felt a deep bitterness. He recalled one occasion in particular in which he himself felt that *the degree to which* he disapproved of the others was disproportionate and that the angry *way in which* he responded to the jokes had made others uneasy.

As a result of his examination, the man was able to see that, like the beaver Arthur, he "had never played anything with anybody" and, moreover, that his strong disapproval of anything "frivolous" (which in this case included both the fable itself and the one beaver's behavior) masked the frustration he felt at not being able to take things lightly.

Notice that the "why" question was the last one to be raised. In our experience, it is almost always true that motives are almost always too diffuse and nebulous to act as the starting point for the process of examination. We are more likely to accurately work out "why" we feel or respond in a given way if we can be helped to see a pattern in terms of when, how often, and who or what triggers that response.

The skillful facilitator tries to get the group members to examine their reactions for themselves, as an almost spontaneous effort. In developmental bibliotherapy, the recognition and examination of deeper issues often will happen with little urging. However, new group members or chronic or very ill mental patients can have difficulty just examining the literal level of the literature or specifying their responses. The bibliotherapist facilitates the process of examination with questions such as: "You said you 'kind of liked' the poem? Can you tell me exactly what it was you liked? Did the sound please you? Could you get a picture in your mind from the description? Is there one line that seems particularly true or special to you? Now that you have chosen the line, can you say more about what it means to you?"

In other cases, members will need help in deciding which of several points they should examine carefully. Or the facilitator will have to concentrate on helping a participant examine and formulate feelings in a coherent way so that he or she will be in control both of the feelings and the responses to them.

Clearly, probing feelings until cognitive awareness emerges can be a subtle and difficult task for both the facilitator and the participant. Furthermore, as we will point out more than once in our discussions of specific strategies, probing can also be dangerous if the therapist has not been both empathic and accurate in analyzing problem areas. The facilitator must also work to ensure that the group as a whole is not victimized by one member's uncontrolled response.

Step Three: Juxtaposition

We have spoken of the recognition of a thought or feeling as the result of the impact of a piece of literature. As this recognition is examined, an additional impression of the subject may emerge—an impression that can change or modify one's first response. Thus, in bibliotherapy, examination may lead to *juxtaposition*—that is, to the act of putting side by side, for purposes of comparison and contrast, two impressions of an object or experience.

The new impression that the participant juxtaposes with his or her original response may be either an image, character, situation, or concept found in the literature itself or a concept or feeling that emerged through the dialogue. In either case, the participant looks at his or her original reaction in light of the new input. Particularly when the original values, situations, concepts, attitudes, or feelings have been relatively unexamined, juxtaposing the old with the new input forces a deeper examination of the issues involved.

Several possible responses can result from this process. Contrasting an established opinion or feeling with a newly presented concept may lead to an affirmation of the original position: "*In the course of defending my position against another viewpoint, I am all the more convinced that I do believe what I said and intend to act on it.*"

It is more likely, however, that some modification will come from the process: "*Things seem a bit different than I had thought of them before. This new view exposes something or adds something I had not really examined up to this point. Now I see more clearly how and why such and such is true.*"

Or the juxtaposition may trigger a recognition that the first idea or sensation was not at all valid: "*Now that I see these two interpretations together, I reflect on my earlier feeling or viewpoint and see that the new way of looking at things is better and more meaningful.*"

In many cases, however, the result will sound something like this: "*Now that I have looked carefully at a couple of ways of feeling and viewing this factor, I need more time and other ways of valuing before I can define the way that is valid for me personally. Other bibliotherapy sessions will be helpful.*"

The insight that comes from the process of juxtaposition is not unique to bibliotherapy. However, interactive bibliotherapy is particularly suited for providing (1) an environment that encourages the process of looking for fresh connections among external stimuli and previously held attitudes and feelings; and (2) the external stimuli themselves.

Literature can act as an agent for examination. Elements in the material itself may correct discrepancies, offer role models, and graphically depict alternatives that the participant can examine and then juxtapose by comparing and contrasting them with his or her personal situation.

Literature corrects discrepancies. A work may contain an element that reveals that a strongly held opinion is based on an incorrect understanding. For example, one professional woman had long considered her mother's gardening and collections of decorative thimbles a perfect example of how the mother was trapped in a traditional role. Instead of expanding her world through discussion of books and ideas, the mother seemed content with activities that did not challenge her. But a reading of Alice Walker's "In Search of Our Mother's Gardens" helped the daughter recognize that these passionately pursued activities might actually indicate a thirst for beauty. She began to reexamine her highly critical attitude toward her mother to see if there were other instances in which the criticism was based more on her own failure to see and understand her mother's motives than on the mother's inadequacy.

Literature offers role-model possibilities. Characters or responses in stories, novels, plays, or narrative poems can serve as role models for new behavior.

For example, in discussing "Grandma's Gumption" by H. L. Marshall, participants will often talk about how they have looked up to someone they knew who—like Grandma—had the ability to act even in times of tribulation. The poem triggers insights into precisely why they find this ability important and into their own behavior under pressure.

In another case, Jean Craighead George's *Julie of the Wolves* offered a model to a group of adolescents. At one point Julie is alone with a pack of wolves on an ice field. She becomes temporarily immobilized by fear. Knowing that she will die if she does not act, she remembers her Eskimo father's advice: "'Change your ways when fear seizes,' he had said, 'for it usually means that you are doing something wrong.'"

A school librarian guided the discussion about Julie and her reactions into an exploration of the kinds of fear the young people in her group had. Some talked about the tough kids from a neighboring school. Others mentioned not wanting to play rough games on the street and being afraid both to play and not to play. Others were concerned about making mistakes, either in the code of the street or in the classroom. Returning to the advice in the book, the participants moved the discussion toward deciding on a strategy beforehand that could be used to cope when they next faced the fear-producing situation. Some strategies were formulated, others were not—but all the participants ended up with more insight into their fears. Notice that the model here was not specific: Julie and her situation were very remote from this urban school. But we often find that the lack of specific mirroring in the literature enhances a work's catalytic potential. Focusing on a child in a totally different culture freed these adolescents to talk about something they usually kept safely hidden. They were able to examine and to juxtapose the *pattern of response* in the story and then to use it as a model for themselves.

Literature graphically depicts alternatives. Bibliotherapy materials can help both clinical and developmental participants look at and deal with some of the many alternatives with which they must cope. We have just seen how the literature can offer role models. But it will not always offer positive models. For example, as participants conjecture on the circumstances that brought about the situation described in John Updike's "Ex-Basketball Player," they can develop a personal insight into the way in which drifting results from an insufficient awareness of the realities of adulthood and a failure to plan ahead.

Step Four: Application to Self

As we have just said, the bibliotherapeutic process cannot stop at juxtaposition. The feelings and concepts that have been recognized, examined, and juxtaposed must now become genuinely experienced. The participants complete the process by engaging in the twin steps of evaluation and integration.

Evaluation calls for a new level of recognition and examination. The participants must look within to become aware of themselves; they must look at how their attitudes and behaviors are affected by their new viewpoints. But if the experience is to be fully therapeutic, they must go beyond cognitive awareness and make a personal commitment to using the new attitudes as a reference point for response or action. In other words, the insights must be *integrated.*

In effect, the self-awareness that has been developing throughout the previous three steps now comes into focus by means of this final step. To use Walker Percy's terminology, the material helps the individuals *name* themselves (Percy 1975). In the traditional forms of psychotherapy, such naming prompts the patients to look within for the initial source of material. Thus, in *The Structure of Magic* (Bandler and Grinder 1975), therapists are told to try renaming what they perceive to have come from within the patients; in other words, they build on the participants' self-generated expressions of their problems or feelings. By the same token, Meichenbaum and Cameron (1974) talk of "the clinical potential of modifying what clients say to themselves."

In bibliotherapy, however, the naming starts from the literature; that is, it begins with a universally applicable expression of a unique viewpoint, experience, or image. The participant thus names another's description but does so through the unique filter of self. The dimension of distance works as a prism, such that the dancing refractions of light upon a screen made up of verbalized "names" and nonverbal body responses can, as it were, be seen and heard—and can, in fact, be renamed—by the participant, the others, and the facilitator. The naming process is enlarged, refined, and, it is hoped, clarified in the bibliotherapeutic dialogue.

The dialogue, which facilitates self-application, continues to refer back to the material. For example, evaluation often involves helping the participants ask themselves such questions as

- How does the concept or situation that has been discussed apply to me?
- How do I deal with feelings that the materials and dialogue have raised? By denial? Or by considering them to be steps toward growth?
- What impact does this reaction have on my life? What do I have to do to integrate the new insight? Am I willing to change?

Both evaluation and making a commitment to change take time. Some clinical group sessions may go on for months or even years before participants show signs of reaching or completing the final step of self-application.

However, the act of repeatedly being asked to look at the literature, to experience and express a feeling-response, and to work toward analyzing and integrating that response may well have some eventual catalytic force.

Although it acts as a reference point for discussion, the literature nonetheless continues to act as a catalyst rather than as the direct focus of self-application. As we have seen in the previous three steps, the process is carried out through dialogue.

Several different kinds of self-awareness might emerge as a result of completing the bibliotherapeutic process. On the one hand, participants come to see the personal force contained in a word or concept. But they also discover that this meaning is both shared *and* different from the meaning experienced by other group members. Through recognition, but also through affirmation of a uniquely personal meaning and understanding, the participants can come to terms with the implications of the feelings for themselves. Ultimately, they can move to more creative, self-utilizing behaviors.

Bibliotherapy as a Process

Thus far we have detailed the four steps in the bibliotherapeutic process. Several additional key features characterize the process as a whole.

Bibliotherapy is continuous

Although the four steps can be distinguished from one another and always follow the same sequence, they neither take place at a uniform rate nor are they necessarily completed during each session; furthermore, the bibliotherapeutic process is continuous. In developmental groups, all four steps can regularly be completed by most of the participants. In the course of a single session, it is even possible that some participants will move from one recognition to another, thereby completing each of the four steps of the process more than once. On the other hand, as in the case of severely regressed patients, the facilitator may be satisfied with helping members achieve some recognition and a minimal amount of examination of an issue or experience.

In other words, in the context of an actual session, the process is not always tidy. Examination and juxtaposition may give rise to a new recognition, which one or another participant begins to examine in turn. And, of course, one group member may quickly move toward self-application while another is still caught up in examination.

The four steps of the bibliotherapeutic process are continuous in yet another important way: All the steps involve the complementary processes of analysis and synthesis.

Analysis. Analysis involves the separating of a feeling or idea into its parts, delving into each component, and, finally, seeing how one part might relate to the whole. In bibliotherapy, the facilitator helps participants dissect both their feelings and the reasons for them so that they can eventually put the factors together in a meaningful way.

In this connection, the bibliotherapist should always begin with analysis of the *conscious material* evoked by the literature and the subsequent dialogue. Certainly such conscious material is the most readily available. In many cases, the individuals can gain a great deal of self-affirmation as well as self-understanding by looking closely at feelings and concepts that are conscious but have not been reflected upon.

At the same time, however, bibliotherapeutic literature—particularly poetry—often has an emotional impact that can release *unconscious material* (i.e., material of which the individual is unaware). In a later chapter we will look at how the skilled and trained bibliotherapist can use such an approach to help members analyze what is significant for their self-awareness without endangering their sense of self-preservation.

Synthesis. The analysis that breaks a thought or concept down into its component parts is often completed or complemented by synthesis. In the latter process, separate materials are combined into a single coherent entity. Thus, in bibliotherapy, the concepts, images, and emotions that have been distinguished are synthesized by a fresh perception of how these diverse elements might fit together. The participants make their own connections among feelings, situations, or concepts that (1) they have recognized as having value, and (2) have been brought up either by the literature itself, by fellow group members, or by the facilitator. All of these elements are synthesized into a fresh way of looking at things. This insight can then be used to reinforce an old way or to create a new solution.

Bibliotherapy is creative

There is much we still do not understand about the role of creativity in therapeutic growth. It does seem, however, that some kind of intimate connection exists between the process of creation and the kind of therapeutic process we have just described. In particular, theories about artistic or scientific creativity seem especially closely related to the step we have called juxtaposition. Again and again, the literature about creativity emphasizes the making of an original *relationship* between two elements, neither of which is necessarily original in itself.

For example, Antony Starr (1972) sees a split between the inner and the outer world; the attempt to bridge this split involves a juxtaposition between the conflicting feelings or ideas. In addition, Albert Rothenberg (1979a, 1979b, 1979c) identifies the creative effort in the conscious thought pattern involved in looking at antithetical elements and producing new entities and creations. In a similar vein, Silvano Arieti (1966, 1967, 1978) notes that the ability to register similarity is a common factor in psychopathology, in creativity, and in normality. The capacity to differentiate similarities among many experiences is so significant that Arieti even attributes to it the ultimate rise and fall of humankind.

Rollo May sees an "encounter" as the critical factor in creativity. He describes what we have termed as "juxtaposition" when he says, "The pole of the world is an inseparable part of the creativity of an individual. What occurs is always a *process*, a *doing*—specifically a process interrelating the person and his or her world" (May 1975, 44–45).

All of these theories developed as a result of the authors' concern with the ways in which artistic and scientific achievements are produced. The process described by these authors, however, is one that can have great *internal significance* without necessarily resulting in an external achievement. Whenever an individual makes a new and unexpected connection among attitudes, feelings, or experiences—a connection that results in personal growth and feeling—that person has engaged in a creative act. Creativity has been exercised even if the viewpoint in question is never translated into a painting, a poem, or a scientific hypothesis. In this sense, the growth in itself is the created product.

In helping participants work out a juxtaposition, the bibliotherapist is facilitating the essential link between the recognition and examination of an idea or feeling and its application to the inner self. In other words, juxtaposition is the creative heart of the bibliotherapeutic process.

Language as a key feature

In bibliotherapy, the creative process cannot be separated from language. In fact, one of the distinguishing features of interactive bibliotherapy is that language serves as both stimulus and agent in the therapeutic process.

In the first place, the *language of the literature* is the catalytic tool that initiates the creative process. One of the advantages involved in using literature as a tool is that some kind of explicit juxtaposition is often present in the material itself. We can allude only briefly here to the dynamics of figurative language, but note that it is the nature of metaphor to create a link between two different, apparently disparate elements. Thus, especially in poetry, the language of the text can provide a vivid and memorable model of how to transfer what is well known to an understanding of what is less well known.

For example, Norma Farber's poem "I'll Know Daybreak" sets up such a juxtaposition very strikingly when she says in the last line that she will know daybreak

When I wake in the morning by choice.

Participants responding to this poem have gotten into heated discussions about the difference each of them sees between the meaning of that line and of one earlier in the poem about waking in the morning "by chance." "Chance" and "choice" are examined carefully, juxtaposed in terms of each participant's private experience, and then applied to self.

Thus, although the language of the literature can be a model, the creative dynamic actually takes place through the *language of the dialogue*. James E. Miller's observations on the power of language in his excellent book, *Word, Self, Reality*, apply to the role that language plays in bibliotherapy:

> In the process of sorting out his thoughts, or of disentangling and examining his tangled experiences, he is in effect defining himself, outlining himself, asserting and proclaiming himself. There can be no more vital activity for the individual: the results and the actions (new thoughts and new experiences) proceeding from it will further define his identity, not only for him but for the world he inhabits. (Miller 1972, 111)

Miller's analysis is another expression of the "naming" process discussed earlier. But his remarks also indicate the important role that communication plays in the bibliotherapeutic process: The self the participant struggles to become aware of is unique and cannot be known by another with certitude unless the participant is willing to share. Through the bibliotherapeutic dialogue, increased self-awareness is often accompanied by self-disclosure. As Sidney Jourard has noted, "No man can come to know himself except as an outcome of disclosing himself to another person (1964, 5)." Or, to use Buber's phrase again, the act of sharing the self can bring about "healing through meeting."

Effectiveness of the Bibliotherapeutic Process

Although bibliotherapists and outside observers alike can testify that the process we have just described has brought about personal growth and enrichment, much can also be learned from formal research that verifies the effectiveness of literature as a tool. Ross (1977) provides an excellent model of a well-conceived research study. Unfortunately, other academic researchers have not always been careful about considered variables such as differences in setting, training of the facilitator, or techniques. In addition, they tend to assume that the therapeutic processes operating in reading bibliotherapy are equivalent to those involved in interactive bibliotherapy. In other words, many researchers have not distinguished between groups in which reading is prescribed and no discussion is held and groups in which a facilitated dialogue is considered central to the process. For example, in their analysis of the effectiveness of bibliotherapy, Schrank and Engels

(1981) consider the two aforementioned approaches to be equivalent. Consequently, their study is of limited use. As this discussion has shown, the procedures, the goals, and, ultimately, the effectiveness of interactive bibliotherapy lie precisely in the facilitated interaction, not in the act of reading.

At the same time, other areas of research that do not identify themselves with bibliotherapy can also illuminate the bibliotherapeutic process. Hence bibliotherapists can find insights in studies (such as that by Rogers [1973]) on the dynamics of metaphor or the effectiveness of imagery. Some of the research on reading and learning, as well, can clarify both what happens in the bibliotherapeutic process and how effective a tool literature is. For example, MacNamee (1985) has studied the impact of storytelling and dramatization on the learning of preschoolers as well as learning-disabled children.

Importance of Strengths in the Bibliotherapeutic Process

One conclusion almost certain to emerge from research is that the emphasis on strengths plays a fundamental role in the bibliotherapeutic process. In the first place, the initiative for each step of the process lies with the participant. The facilitator can guide, but it is the individual participant who must recognize, examine, juxtapose, and integrate the feeling-responses and the understandings. Of course, the capacity to take the initiative is a fundamentally healthy act. Moreover, progression from the first to the final step calls increasingly on the individual's strengths. As indicated in the earlier discussion of goals, the first step of simple recognition means that the participant has some positive capacity to relate to objects and experiences outside the self. However, if the participant is to be able to genuinely integrate an insight, he or she must exercise a whole network of positive qualities, including (1) some ability to analyze issues, (2) sufficient honesty to look at the inner self, (3) enough objectivity to view a feeling or behavior pattern from another perspective, and, finally, (4) adequate self-confidence and hope to feel that change is possible and that one is personally capable of making such a change.

Another way of making the same point is to say again that bibliotherapy is a process of *self-actualization*. Moreover, we consider the self-actualizing process to be one that not only enhances existing strengths but also corrects discrepancies. Thus it is therapeutic for one individual to realize that her strong sense of isolation comes less from active rejection by others than from her own unwillingness to share her feelings. But equally growth producing is a dialogue that helps another person see himself more clearly as someone who is willing to extend himself to others.

There is another closely related dimension to the role of "strengths" in the bibliotherapeutic process. We have said that the outcome of this process is growth. In its turn, growth can be evaluated in terms of two quite different perspectives. On the one hand, we can see it as a corrective process in which deficiencies or inadequacies have been overcome, developmental lags have been successfully bridged, and discrepancies have been corrected.

But we prefer to see a positive understanding of growth as a process that should be evaluated in terms of how well desirable qualities are developed and reinforced. In this sense, the strengths are both *a necessary part of the process* and *the significant measure of the result.* We might note here that others in the mental health field such as Buber (1963, 1970), Erikson (1964), Jahoda (1958), Otto (1963, 1965, 1968a, 1968b, 1979), Shostrom (1976), and Maslow (1970, 1971a, 1971b) also prefer to emphasize strengths.

The discussion in this handbook will necessarily return again and again to the issue of strengths. Coverage will include such matters as the utilization, development, and facilitation of various strengths during the course of a bibliotherapy session, as well as the specific strengths to be measured in the context of a participant's responses.

STUDY GUIDE

1. Summarize the four steps of the bibliotherapeutic process. Include a brief definition of each step.

2. Write a brief statement in which you explain your understanding of literature as a useful tool in bibliotherapy. If your background includes teaching or mental health work, you can develop a comparison between that mode and bibliotherapy.

3. Look up one of the following general studies of creativity: Starr (1972), Rothenberg (1979a, 1979b, 1979c), Kubie (1961, 137–143), May (1975, 1–45), Maslow (1967, 1971a, 1971b), a section from one of Arieti's discussions of creativity and mental health (1966, 1967, 1978), or one essay from the collections edited either by Austin (1978), Parnes and Harding (1962), or Rothenberg and Hausman (1976). In addition, read one of the following discussions of creativity and the "creative therapies": Burns (1977), Heninger (1977), D. K. Miller (1978), Silverman (1973), Vaccaro (1979), Zwerling (1979), or Berry (1977). Next, briefly analyze, compare, and contrast the two theories you have selected; then write out your view of the relationship of these theories of creativity to bibliotherapy.

4. Analyze Miller's statement on language, quoted in the section entitled "Language as a key feature," and relate it to the place of language in bibliotherapy. Recognize that this is an exploratory statement. Your understanding of this point will change as you become more experienced.

5. Comment on your understanding of the importance of strengths to the bibliotherapeutic process. Use specific examples. If you are not clear about the qualities that constitute strengths, refer to Chapter 11 as well as to the sources given in "Further Readings."

PRACTICUM

1. Choose an item for bibliotherapeutic use and indicate, line by line, how *you* would respond in terms of the four-step process described in this chapter. In doing this exercise, you are simulating the steps involved in a developmental bibliotherapy session.

2. Use a poem to show the differences among a feeling-response, cognitive awareness, and an integrated response.

3. Answer the "Self-Disclosure Questionnaire" (Jourard 1964, 159–164) to further your own self-knowledge. Think through and answer each question as fully as you can. Sharpen your sense of the differences between writing out self-disclosing statements and expressing them aloud by answering some questions in writing and recording others. Note the feelings that arise as you do both, just as you must recall your own hesitations and difficulties in formulating your responses during an actual bibliotherapy session. Such reflections should help you better understand the participants.

FURTHER READINGS

The following studies on emotion offer valuable background. Ekman (1972) and Izard (1977) provide good general material, and Gaylin (1979, 195–302) has a chapter on "Feeling Moved," which applies to feeling responses in bibliotherapy. Sorokin (1950) offers a series of essays on the importance of strengths, including the writings of Allport, Sorokin, Duchesne, and Greenblatt. Goble (1971, 119–142) provides an insightful analysis of Maslow's thoughts on the importance of personal strengths. Jahoda (1958, 22–64) develops criteria for positive mental health. Miller's (1972) work is not about bibliotherapy as such, but it illuminates the dynamics of the dialogue and of the creative writing process. Rosenblatt (1978) does not confuse the personal process with the dialogic component in bibliotherapy. She has much of value to say in her chapters entitled "Efferent and Esthetic Reading" and "Interpretation, Evaluation, and Criticism." Finally, Bleich (1975) offers an interesting and valuable analysis of subjective criticism.

— PART 2 —

LITERATURE: THE TOOL OF BIBLIOTHERAPY

4

Criteria for Choosing Bibliotherapeutic Materials

A bibliotherapist came across an anthology of poetry by F. H. Willette entitled Shadows and Light. *She decided to scan the collection for poems she might add to her files for use in future bibliotherapy sessions. In the next hour, despite two phone calls and a problem about the next day's schedule, she managed to evaluate the potential of the thirty-five poems for bibliotherapeutic use.*

Overall, she felt it was advantageous that most of the poems used imagery from nature and everyday life and that the rhythm and rhyme were also generally effective. Even so, as she skimmed through the book, she concluded that many of the poems would not quite work as bibliotherapy material.

For example, she briefly considered one called "Quack Grass," which began

> *There's very little can be done*
> *For gardens under-webbed by quack.*
> *All one can do is curse it well*
> *And cut it back.*

She was interested by this poem's theme of the troublesome issues in life that cause conflict and must somehow be rooted out. But she also found that the phrasing and word choice necessitated a bit of work to grasp the image. In the bibliotherapist's experience, many participants would end up puzzling over the vocabulary and diction instead of experiencing a spontaneous feeling-response. At the same time, the connection between quack grass (i.e., weeds) and human affairs was not articulated but, rather, was left implicit. Consequently, the theme was likely to escape those literal-minded participants who had difficulty understanding metaphors. She concluded that she was not likely to use this piece with a group.

However, she then came to another poem on a related theme. Entitled "Quarrel," this one began

> Your voice blows chill as wintry gales
> And mine in answer rasps like nails
> Across a blackboard. With your eyes
> My eyes contend for ego's prize.

She immediately sensed that this poem had much more potential—the phrasing was easier to follow, and the similes made it easy to see the connection between image and theme. The bibliotherapist also liked the light tone that kept the resolution from sounding too preachy or pat. Since she needed poems that dealt well with the theme of quarrels and conflict, she decided to add this poem to her files.

As she continued to page through the collection, the bibliotherapist found more examples in which the language, imagery, or treatment were problematic in terms of the criteria she was using. For example, coming as she did from a farm background, the bibliotherapist personally was moved by several poems that dealt with rural life; yet she was aware that the themes were not really universal enough to use with the participants from urban backgrounds with whom she worked.

However, there was one poem that she found very striking, even though she felt, once again, that some participants might find its allusiveness and language difficult. Entitled "Eve to Cain," the poem went

> O wild and wilful son, conceived in grief
> And birthed in pain, small wonder woman's chiding
> Stayed not your hand; but know with full belief
> Where'er you dwell in savage exiled hiding,
> That of the twain who nurtured at my breast
> I loved slain Abel's darkling brother best.

Several times she had felt that the participants in the chemically dependent group needed more selections dealing with parental rejection. Therefore, even though this poem seemed to be directed to a very specific audience, she marked it for inclusion in her files.

In the end, then, although there were many poems in this collection that pleased her personally, the bibliotherapist concluded that only two *or possibly three of the thirty-five could actually be added to her files for use as bibliotherapy material.*

TIME AND AGAIN, BIBLIOTHERAPISTS looking for material have the kind of experience we have just described: For every piece of literature that is added to the files, many more are found to be unsuitable for one reason or another. Although bibliotherapeutic and literary criteria are not incompatible, the bibliotherapist must distinguish between good poetry on the one hand and material that experience indicates would be a good tool for therapeutic discussion on the other.

The qualities that a bibliotherapist looks for can be broken down into four thematic and four stylistic dimensions. The following table summarizes the spectrum of qualities in each dimension, with the most desirable ones on the left and the least desirable on the right.

Thematic Dimensions

Universal experience or emotion		Personalized
Powerful		Trite
Comprehensible		Obscure
Positive	(Ambiguous)	Negative

Stylistic Dimensions

Compelling rhythm	Sing-song/discontinuous rhythm
Imagery	Imagery
striking	hackneyed or absent
concrete	abstract
Language	Language
simple, precise vocabulary	difficult or archaic vocabulary
clear, simple diction	convoluted diction
Complexity	Complexity
manageable length	long
succinct	diffuse, rambling

We will discuss each of these dimensions in some detail, with examples. Note that although many of the works mentioned in the discussion are poems, the criteria can and should be applied to other forms of material. Furthermore, we will indicate any special considerations that apply to a specific genre in a given dimension.

Thematic Considerations

In general, the thematic dimensions are more important than the stylistic ones. Only rarely, for example, would a bibliotherapist decide that the stylistic values of a work outweigh thematic weakness. On the other hand, one regularly comes across a work whose language or form seems problematic but whose message is just right for a particular group or individual.

Universal themes. There is no conflict between aesthetic standards and the first thematic dimension. Both good literature and literature good for bibliotherapy have *universal themes*—that is, they treat emotions and experiences that can be readily identified and identified with.

In previous chapters, we have already named a number of works that seem to be able to touch virtually everyone. For example, a poem like Sandburg's "Soup," or the Hassidic tale that opens this book, deals with emotions and experiences that are fundamental to the human condition and could be discussed by virtually any population.

However, as we saw earlier in the bibliotherapist's choice of "Eve to Cain," there are experiences and emotions that are deeply meaningful to a more restricted group. If such a theme is presented effectively, the work should be used with the appropriate group.

The bottom line for evaluating universality is the decision as to whether the subject or theme is presented in such a way that it remains part of the writer's personal world rather than an experience with which another can identify. In other words, if there is nothing in the poem with any real potential for stimulating recognition, the work is unlikely to sustain the other three steps of the bibliotherapeutic process.

Powerful themes. It is not enough for a work to have a universal theme, however. That theme must also be presented in such a way that it becomes *powerful* rather than trite. Actually the distinction between powerful and universal is somewhat elusive. But, basically, we are trying to indicate that it is critical for a work to touch the participants in a vital way. This is not to say that the theme of the work must communicate something that *everyone knows* but, rather, that it should say something in such a way that *each one feels,* on the basis of his or her individual history, that what is said has some personal truth or meaning.

Almost every adult, for example, has had an experience that brings home the point made in W. H. Auden's "Musée des Beaux Arts": One person's suffering takes place "while someone else is eating or opening a window or just dully walking along." But the effectiveness of this poem does not come just from the fact that it describes a universal experience. It comes from the way the poet concretely establishes the contrast between the tremendous significance of birth, pain, and death for those experiencing them and the trivial activities that others are pursuing at the same moment in time.

A theme couched in vague, general terms without a sharp image to give it meaning is unlikely to stimulate the participant to explore the *personal* implications of the thought. By the same token, a work that offers an unrealistic, oversimplified moral denies the complexity and intensity of emotions that the bibliotherapist hopes to help the participants confront and deal with. Thus, a poem like Henry Wadsworth Longfellow's "The Rainy Day" urges acceptance of the reality that

> *into each life some rain must fall,*
> *some days must be dark and dreary.*

But the poem offers nothing but sheer willpower as an aid in the difficult process of working out a healthy resignation. In this case, most participants will find little to say in terms of personal evaluation, once they agree or disagree with the platitude.

Here we are discussing specifically the criteria applied by the *bibliotherapist* when selecting literature. When group members are invited to bring in material, some may bring in a saccharine verse from a greeting card or some other trite item. Rather than reject such an offering the bibliotherapist should draw out what made the work seem of value to that individual. In this instance, the focus of the discussion might well be to help the participant see the inadequacy or trivial character of the message. In some cases, the individual may even recognize that the tendency to cling to simplistic answers has interfered with his or her ability to cope with reality.

One other confusion should be avoided in evaluating the power of a theme. There is a critical difference between a work that *is simplistic* and one that *has simplicity.* Many very powerful poems do not look that impressive at first glance: Four to six lines long, they use simple language without innovative techniques. Nonetheless, they somehow make a point that is incredibly complex and fruitful. Robert Frost and Langston Hughes are both masters of such simple explosions. For example, the simile that "Life ain't no crystal stair" in Hughes's "Mother to Son" is easy to grasp, but it exposes the full complexity of the theme we just saw simplistically stated by Longfellow.

In other cases, the line between what is simplistic and what is simple may not be obvious. For example, Lois Lenski's "People" may seem to be limited in both insight and execution, yet this verse has nearly always stimulated a good discussion in both clinical and developmental groups. That is, virtually every participant is likely to know a specific tall person, or a thin one, and thus can initiate a response to this poem. What comes clear as the dialogue goes on, of course, is that everyone can profit from recognizing or reaffirming that the world is made up of many different sorts and that it really is a good thing that we are not all alike.

In the end, the surest way to determine which works are productively simple and which are overly simplistic is to build up experience—and to get the most out of that experience by keeping good records.

Comprehensible themes. Basically, there is little difference in the first two thematic dimensions betwen bibliotherapeutic and aesthetic standards. But the other two criteria for judging the thematic potential of material for bibliotherapy really do reflect the distinct goals of bibliotherapy. If a work is to be a successful catalyst for therapeutic discussion, its theme must be easily *comprehended* by the individual participants. Many fine works are too obscure for use in a bibliotherapy session, for several reasons. First, even though the theme of a work may be universal, the participants may not identify with the image(s) through which it is communicated. Poems or stories from earlier periods of history or from restricted subcultures, for example, might depend heavily on images or experiences that are not part of most peoples' lives.

Second, the theme may not be explicit enough. As we saw in the bibliotherapist's consideration of the poem "Quack Grass," some individuals and populations operate in very literal terms; they are not able to work out a metaphor for themselves, especially when they do not have much experience with imaginative concepts. Note that there is no single standard that can be applied to all populations. For example, developmental and chemically dependent group members tend rather quickly to pick up the habit of looking beyond the immediate meaning. But metaphors make some people uneasy, and others never really become capable of the kind of abstraction that is called for by a complex metaphor; some clinical groups, for example, will be able to understand only those works in which the imagery is concrete and explicitly spelled out.

Third, the theme of a work may be very complex and diffuse, or it may deal with an abstract concept that is hard to distill into a readily identifiable statement about emotion or experience. Thus, works by poets like Lowell, Yeats, or Eliot—who depend on a strong intellectual element—are often not suitable for bibliotherapy.

Clearly, then, the nature of the group for whom the material is being chosen must be considered in making judgments about how comprehensible a work is. Nonetheless, as a general rule we have found that the main idea of an effective selection should be grasped almost immediately, as therapeutic responses tend to be diffused if the participants begin by intellectualizing about the meaning of the material.

Furthermore, although participants will often have a copy of the text to refer to, their spontaneous response really comes from the impact of what they have *heard*. Even if they are being attentive, group members must listen through such predictable distractions as shuffling of papers, shifting of bodies, or noises from outside the meeting room. Therefore, we have found it useful to evaluate materials in a somewhat distracting atmosphere, such as that described in the opening vignette. If the facilitator can see potential in such circumstances, the item is more likely to have meaning and impact when read with the participants.

Nonetheless, the facilitator may deliberately decide to use a difficult work. For example, although the first few lines of Auden's "Musée des Beaux Arts" are fairly clear, the rest of the poem builds on veiled allusions to specific paintings by Brueghel in the Brussels art museum. Such allusions require a more demanding procedure than is usually desirable for bibliotherapeutic material. Still, the theme is so universal and the treatment so powerful that the poem has been used successfully with both developmental and clinical groups. Particularly in clinical groups, we sometimes offset the difficulties of the piece by having the group examine a reproduction of Brueghel's painting of Icarus just before or after the reading.

However, note again that the point of the dialogue is not to further understanding of the references in the poem so much as it is to help the participants deal with what the point made about suffering means to them personally. Some will come to see that the indifference to suffering described in Auden's poem is an almost universal reality, not a personal rejection that necessarily indicates ill-will toward the individual. The dialogue in this case may turn to ways that other participants have found to deal with the isolation that suffering often involves. Or if the participants are not ready to look at psychic suffering, the facilitator can help them look at different responses to physical pain.

Positive themes. The last thematic dimension involves an evaluation of the degree to which a work is *positive* and offers hope. This criterion is central to an overall understanding of bibliotherapy. At the same time, however, we must be clear about exactly how we see this dimension.

In the first place, this criterion is not related to issues of literary merit. Many good pieces of literature are angry, negative, and even despairing. But such works will do little to further the goals of bibliotherapy—namely, to affirm the strengths of the participants, to improve their self-esteem, and/or to help them deal more creatively with their lives, particularly with realities that they cannot change.

On the one hand, a work with a strongly negative tone is likely to feed or bring to the surface feelings of anxiety, inadequacy, and hopelessness. Think, for example, of the well-known poem by Edwin Arlington Robinson entitled "Richard Cory." Its theme is unquestionably universal, powerful, and comprehensible. But its conclusion—that Richard Cory, for all his enviable wealth and status, "one calm summer night, went home and put a bullet through his head"—is far too negative to be suitable for most bibliotherapy sessions. As real as anger, envy, despair, and suicidal impulses may be, they are also fundamentally destructive. Robinson's poem offers neither any resolution nor any hint of how to cope successfully with such feelings. There is nothing healthy about the message, nor is the discussion of it likely to take a therapeutic focus. Rather, it is likely to stir up powerful, threatening emotions that the facilitator will have difficulty dealing with or following up adequately in most group situations.

Admittedly, a skilled and empathic facilitator working with an individual might use this material in a one-on-one setting in which the therapeutic dialogue would emphasize the futility of Cory's solution and move on to dealing with positive ways of coping with the negative emotions that make suicide tempting. In any case, experience is the best guide for judging whether a particular work is too negative for a given individual or situation or whether a carefully facilitated dialogue about the piece could prove therapeutic.

A second distinction is in order here. The bibliotherapeutic material can be used to expose and vent negative feelings. But the work itself should not suggest that a negative solution or reaction is inevitable; nor should it encourage the blocking of a change of attitude. Rather, good bibliotherapeutic material will help identify negative feelings in a way that will lead to liberating action, particularly if the participant develops some insight into the nature of his or her feelings and, as a result, begins to understand how to tolerate the unpleasant reality or to shift the crippling attitude or coping pattern.

But our emphasis on works with positive thematic elements should not be taken for a recommendation of items with a Pollyanna attitude. As we indicated in the section entitled "Powerful themes," the bibliotherapist is just as mistaken in offering an unrealistic or oversimplified message as in offering a despairing one. Realistic hope and affirmation do not trivialize real suffering and struggle, nor do they suggest that a smile will cure all woes or that with proper management everyone can live happily ever after.

Ambiguity

In fact, it is likely that many poems with high bibliotherapeutic potential will be fairly ambiguous. This very ambiguity may become an important factor during the discussion phase. What one person sees as grim may seem somewhat hopeful to another or even liberating to a third. As the different reactions emerge, participants have a direct experience of the fact that a given event or feeling is not always understood in the same way. Indeed, seeing a quite different reaction may free an individual to change a response that previously seemed to be the only one possible. The ambiguity of the material, which invites such varying responses, may well help bibliotherapy participants understand a very critical point of good mental health—that one's personal *reaction* to the realities of life can change, even if the realities themselves do not.

Humor

The problem of ambiguity touches on some of the same issues involved in using humorous material in bibliotherapy. We saw how the bibliotherapist looking through the Willette collection approved the light touch in "Quarrel" because it kept a serious point from being made too absolutely or too somberly. Her reaction reflects the kind of thinking that led Moody in *Laugh After Laugh* (1978) to conclude that there is a strong case for supporting the relationship between a sense of humor and good mental health.

Laughter certainly can indicate a healthy capacity to distance oneself from an issue. Moreover, be it a smile or a belly laugh, the expression of a humorous reaction sets off a physical response, including specific muscular reactions. The experience of Norman Cousins (1979), who credits laughter with relieving the painful symptoms of a very serious illness, has led to some serious exploration of the use of laughter in medicine and mental health.

There is no question that a light touch can open up deep issues, whereas a solemn treatment might make participants uneasy and inhibited. The first response to the Beatles' song, "When I'm 64," may be a smile, but whether or not love will endure is a serious concern for most of us. The song touches on important facets of the issue in a way that is much less threatening—and potentially more revealing—than the blunt query, "How do you feel about long-term commitments?"

Humor is also an excellent vehicle for expressing ambivalence or creating a healthy distance. Members of a women's or parenting group may chuckle appreciatively at Garrison Keillor's interview of the fairytale Gretel in his essay, "My Stepmother, Myself," but they are also likely to gain a new perspective on family relationships. Similarly, the bibliotherapist might decide to use a comic strip like "Cathy" or "Peanuts" as a succinct and wry way to warm up or wrap up a session.

Yet problems may arise when the facilitator begins to evaluate humorous works as bibliotherapy material. On the one hand, good humor often depends on incongruity or irony, both of which call for a certain kind of abstraction. As we saw in the case of metaphors, some bibliotherapy participants may be too literal to understand the meaning that is being implied. Alternatively, the very distancing on which incongruity and irony play may require the bibliotherapist to work hard to keep the dialogue focused on the *personal* implications of the situation and to ensure that the serious side of the theme is not lost. In still other cases, the humor of a piece may depend on an unexpected reversal. A joke of this sort may be funny enough to be used as a warm-up exercise to break the ice or to relax the group but, in itself, is not likely to sustain the kind of scrutiny that bibliotherapeutic discussion calls for.

There is, of course, a whole realm of humor that plays on anger and negative feelings. But works based on such humor are seldom suitable for bibliotherapy because of their fundamentally negative stance. Sarcasm, for instance, depends on belittling or mocking something or someone and is contrary to the attitude of respect for the integrity and rights of others, which is an important part of bibliotherapy. Specific circumstances may arise in which a skillfully facilitated discussion of such material might be useful. In general, however, the bibliotherapist should avoid sarcastic pieces as well as works characterized by a decidedly negative outlook.

In short, although it would be a serious mistake to rule out humorous material altogether, the bibliotherapist must carefully consider the nature of the humor in a given piece in the process of evaluating its potential for therapeutic discussion.

Stylistic Dimensions

As it is not possible to divorce theme from style, there will be some overlap as we discuss what the bibliotherapist looks for in terms of rhythm, imagery, language, and complexity. As was true for the thematic criteria, two of the four stylistic dimensions reflect standards similar to those used by literary critics; the other two, however, reflect the unique goals of bibliotherapy.

Rhythm

Much more work needs to be done on the dynamics of the human response to rhythm. Whether we feel some primordial echo of the rhythm of our mother's heartbeat from the womb (Meerlo 1969), whether we are comforted by the tonal reflection of the rhythms in nature, or whether some other factor is operating, there is no question that *compelling rhythm* makes a work more powerful. Rhythm, often pronounced in poetry or song, is present as well in well-written prose. Films, too, combine word and visual image—in addition to sound—into discernible rhythms.

When a poem falls into a trite da-da-da-da-da, or when a writer depends heavily on a series of short and choppy subject-verb-object sentences, the impact of the content is diminished. In such cases the participant's capacity to attend to the material is apparently disrupted when the sheer sound of it is unattractive. Conversely, clinical and developmental participants alike experience a healthy uplift and sense of delight from the wonderful rhythm of a work like Edgar Allan Poe's "Bells" or Robert Southey's "The Cataract of Lodore." Rhythm alone has been observed to lift deeply depressed and introverted persons out of their private worlds—at least momentarily—and to release memories that later became the basis of therapeutic discussion.

We should note here that those who use remotivation techniques are encouraged to find rhythmic and light verse as introductory material. But remotivation is not meant to be a separate creative arts therapy in itself, as is bibliotherapy. The goals of remotivation are specifically oriented toward helping people focus on practical issues such as "who, why, where, and when" as a function of acquiring communication skills (Pullinger 1960; Robinson n.d.). Remotivation does not share the bibliotherapeutic focus on feeling-responses or imaginative stimulation.

Imagery

The bibliotherapist and the literary critic mean the same thing when they say the imagery should be effective; in other words, it should be striking and concrete rather than trite and abstract. Especially in poetry, the meaning of a work is often carried by the images. Good writers do not merely state what is seen and felt and meant; they present the object or experience in such a way that the reader or listener mentally imagines or remembers what is being described.

But good images are not just comprehensible—they are "telling." They stimulate some *insight* into the nature of the object or scene, or, by extension, into the nature of experience. Imagery helps us assimilate our understanding, not just intellectualize it.

Thus, "I Think I Understand," a popular song from the 1970s by Joni Mitchell, uses imagery to suggest and clarify both fear and the overcoming of fear. The chorus refers to fear as a "wilderland," an invented word that brings up an effective cluster of associations—wild, wilderness, bewilder, wonderland—and the images in each of the verses continue to mix positive and negative associations. There are, for example, images of daylight on the path, forests blocking the way, the path climbing up the hill, the night of fear. The contrast between hope and fear is developed further by the contrast in the refrain between "stepping stones" and "sinking sand." The images are thus both striking and concrete; moreover, they offer a rich source of concepts and feelings to be recognized, explored, accepted, or rejected by the inner self. (By contrast, an image that is shopworn or general may not have even the slightest impact. No one will bother to visualize the specific features or coloring of someone described, say, as "pretty as a picture.")

In short, good bibliotherapeutic material most often contains concrete images of objects found in nature or things and experiences that are part of daily life. As we have noted again and again, a good concrete image can enable the participant to emerge from his or her closed world and focus on some external reality—a stone, a rainbow, one's hands. Yet concrete images need not be strictly literal. Imaginative associations can effectively be made through metaphor and simile. For example, Robert Nathan's "I Ride the Great Black Horses of My Heart" uses a vivid metaphor to suggest the powerful sense of despair the speaker struggles with before he brings his "horses home."

In addition, works that combine imagery with first-person pronouns (I, we, me, us, my, mine, ours) and deal directly with feelings are particularly likely to be successful. On the literal level, the participants are drawn into the kind of personal feeling-responses and associations that bibliotherapy calls for.

Linguistic considerations

Since the bibliotherapeutic material is a catalyst for discussion rather than the primary focus, both the vocabulary and the diction of literature must be *clear.* Thus, on the strength of vocabulary alone, many very fine works of literature are judged to be unsuitable for bibliotherapy. But a very fine line is involved. On the one hand, precise words with strong connotations contribute to good imagery and, as such, are desirable in bibliotherapy materials. On the other, we have seen how important it is that the literature not be so obscure or difficult that many people would need a dictionary to be sure of its meaning. One or two words in a strong story or poem can be explained, of course. And at other times, the context will help clarify the meaning. But in general, if the work cannot be understood by a given group without a review of its difficult or archaic vocabulary, the facilitator should find another piece of material.

We stress this point because the vocabulary of the material can have an impact on the participant's self-esteem and, consequently, on his or her capacity for dialogue. Indeed, the experience of struggling with selections whose language is too difficult can demoralize and/or intimidate those who feel insecure about their ability to learn—and in such cases the literature becomes another sign of inadequacy rather than a tool for affirmation. Even if morale were not an issue, the *feeling*-response to any work that demands an excessive degree of *intellectual* grappling is often sacrificed or at least disrupted.

Even a simple vocabulary can be a bit obtuse, especially when the author has chosen to experiment with syntax (i.e., the grammatical structure of the language). Many participants have trouble, for example, with the way in which e.e. cummings breaks up sentences, phrases, and even words into unusual units or combinations. On the other hand, the syntax need not be so elaborately manipulated to be confusing. Children, participants who have a limited education, and clinical patients who have short attention spans cannot follow long, complex sentences. They are also likely to have trouble with inverted patterns in which not until the end of the sentence is the verb revealed (as in this sentence!).

Clearly, then, bibliotherapists must look carefully at both the vocabulary and the syntax of the material they are evaluating. The fact is that linguistic qualities may well undercut the therapeutic potential of many very fine works of literature for many participants.

Complexity

Stylistic complexity pertains to both the mechanical issue of length and the more elusive problem of structure. For the most part, the best material is *short*. A bibliotherapy session must allow time for presentation of the literature, reflection on it, and full discussion of it. Clearly, a long piece would likely take so much time to present and initially digest that there would be no time left over for discussion. It might also offer so many different stimuli that the participants would be overwhelmed and unable to focus usefully. Accordingly, as it is desirable for each participant to have a copy of the literature to refer to, the material should run no longer than one or two pages of text. Often even a four- to ten-line poem will be evocative enough to sustain a full session.

However, complexity is not always a question of length. A variety of techniques (including allusions, complex interlocking of images, intentional digressions, emphasis on implied rather than explicit meanings) may make a work dense and hard to understand rather than *succinct*. Again, however, the dimension of complexity is judged in terms that have nothing to do with literary value. Instead, the question is whether the work will have the immediate impact that characterizes effective material for interactive bibliotherapy.

It may seem that poems are the only kind of material likely to be appropriately short and succinct. Yet there are a number of prose forms very suitable for bibliotherapy. Fables, myths, and parables often run to no more than a typewritten page or two. Moreover, because they tend to draw on universal images and reflect beliefs about the nature of things, these works can be very powerful tools.

On the other hand, most short stories, essays, and novels cannot be presented as a whole and discussed in a single session. But the facilitator can render them usable by extracting key passages. In developmental groups, the participants might even contract to do some of the reading ahead of time.

Alternatively, some works, particularly nonfiction ones, may be suited to reading in short segments over a number of sessions. Otherwise, a group might work scene by scene through the entire text of a play or simply concentrate on a single passage. Any such extract, of course, should be chosen on the basis of its fulfillment of thematic and stylistic criteria.

Although it is easy to play one song or selection from a record or tape, both length and complexity are factors to be considered when films are the bibliotherapeutic material being used. A film cannot run more than ten to twenty minutes if discussion is to be included within the hour. Faced even with this restriction, however, facilitators have a wide range of possibilities to choose from. Some public libraries have film collections that include short silent films, evocative nature films, educational shorts, and either dramatized or animated versions of traditional tales and legends.

In addition, the increasing popularity of video-recorders makes possible a comprehensive collection of specially edited clips from films and television shows. For example, a discussion could be built around Yoda's discussion of the qualities needed by a Jedi knight in "The Empire Strikes Back," or around the scene in Woody Allen's "Broadway Danny Rose" in which Allen and the Mia Farrow character compare their attitudes about feeling guilty.

Of course, no film or selection should be presented until it has been carefully evaluated by the facilitator for its potential impact. In particular, works that rely on flashbacks or use a loose, impressionistic treatment may be too difficult or diffuse for use with many bibliotherapy participants.

Applying the Criteria

We offer these thematic and stylistic dimensions as general guides. If you are a beginner who is trying to build up files of usable materials, you should discipline yourself to work out ratings for individual works. By forcing yourself to be precise about what adds to or detracts from the bibliotherapeutic potential of a given work, you will focus and sharpen your evaluative skills. It might be helpful, for instance, to develop a record form on which a given work could be rated in each dimension on a scale from one to five, with the highest number indicating the highest potential in that dimension.

As you become more experienced, however, you will find that no rating system is absolute. Most people can agree on which works have very high potential and which are totally inappropriate. Most selections, however, fall somewhere in between. In the final analysis, there is no sure-fire formula for distinguishing a mediocre work that is potentially effective from one that is entirely unviable. (The present authors, for example, have gone ahead with poems that may otherwise have seemed much too difficult and intellectual, and found that they did stir a profound discussion for a given group. And, of course, some works that looked ideal for our bibliotherapeutic use simply fell flat.)

In short, judgments about these dimensions will always have a subjective element. For example, a group of bibliotherapists once found they had totally different estimates of how to rate Dylan Thomas's "Do Not Go

Gentle into That Good Night" in terms of the fourth thematic dimension. One facilitator saw this poem as decidedly negative and likely to feed an unhealthy refusal to accept death. Others felt that the message was at least ambiguous, if not a positive encouragement to live life to the fullest. As the discussion went on, it became clear the one facilitator's judgment primarily reflected her own positive attitude toward life after death. All agreed that this was not a good poem for her to use since her own response to it was so strong that she might have had trouble facilitating very different reactions. The principle suggested here is a good one to follow in general: If something about the theme or style of a particular work seems jarring, use another piece. Not surprisingly, you will find it easier to facilitate material with which you are personally comfortable.

Gauging the Potential of Bibliotherapeutic Materials

Up to this point, we have concentrated on how well a given piece of material is likely to work as a tool for bibliotherapy. In other words, we have looked at criteria for determining whether or not a work has potential for acting as a catalyst for therapeutic discussion and thus for furthering the overall goals of bibliotherapy.

But we have not yet considered how to gauge exactly how the goals are likely to be met through use of a given work. As we have indicated, the discussion of a good selection can go in any one of several directions and is likely to serve more than one major goal or one aspect of that goal. By the same token, it is unlikely that a single work will serve all goals equally well in all respects.

Specific objectives

The following list gives specific objectives for each of the four major therapeutic goals of bibliotherapy. We have formulated the objectives so that they can be used to gauge the specific kind of enrichment and responses that are likely to develop from discussion of a particular work.

I. Goal: The work improves the capacity to respond by stimulating and enriching mental images and feelings that:
   Objective 1: Encourge verbalization and written responses
   Objective 2: Increase awareness of nature
      a. Geographical aspects (mountains, rivers, deserts, seas)
      b. Growing things (plants, animals)
      c. Tactile qualities (textures, hardness, softness)
      d. Seasons (factual and symbolic implications)

Objective 3: Increase awareness of sounds and silence
Objective 4: Increase awareness of visual images and color
Objective 5: Increase awareness of tastes and smells
Objective 6: Increase awareness of touch
Objective 7: Open up the imagination

II. Goal: The work enhances the value of personhood and helps the participant more accurately perceive the self by:
Objective 1: Providing images of the human body
Objective 2: Emphasizing the significance of the human body
Objective 3: Exposing attitudes and feelings about self
Objective 4: Stimulating emotions, feelings, and moods (including healthy humor)
Objective 5: Increasing awareness of processes of growth, change in nature and in self, and in time itself
Objective 6: Stirring memories
Objective 7: Increasing awareness of chemical dependency as it relates to self

III. Goal: The work enlightens interpersonal relationships by increasing awareness of:
Objective 1: The effect of altruism or selfishness
Objective 2: Love and friendship or their absence
Objective 3: Anger, jealousy, and hatred
Objective 4: Dealing with frustration or success
Objective 5: Chemical dependency as it influences others
Objective 6: Communication (listening and sharing) and understanding others
Objective 7: Family relationships
Objective 8: Responsibility to others

IV. Goal: The work enlarges reality-orientation to the world we live in by increasing awareness of:
Objective 1: Everyday tools of living
Objective 2: Life-style and its meaning
Objective 3: Work
Objective 4: Leisure
Objective 5: Life and its meaning
Objective 6: Death and its meaning
Objective 7: Adversity
Objective 8: Well-being and strengths

Applying the gauges

Perhaps the best way to explain how the gauges can be used is to look at how they would be applied to a specific work. Robert Frost's "Stopping by a Woods on a Snowy Evening" has strong potential for use as a tool for a bibliotherapy discussion: It offers a powerful, basically positive treatment of a universal theme, presented in terms that are immediately comprehensible. In stylistic terms, the compelling rhythm, striking images, simple language, and succinct presentation make the poem ideal for use with almost any group.

But precisely what directions might be taken in the dialogue about this work? The strong concrete images of the poem make it very suitable for a discussion designed to meet the first four objectives under the first major goal—improving the capacity to respond. Objective 1 could be served by having members talk about their own responses to a snowy day; or, if the discussion made it appropriate, the session might end by having each member jot down a list of personal "promises to keep." The references to the wood and lake could well stimulate images of nature (Objective 2). They may also provide an excellent stimulus for considering sound and silence (Objective 3) and visual images (Objective 4). However, this particular poem is not oriented directly toward sensations of touch or taste, nor does it especially encourage use of the imagination.

Some of the objectives under the second major goal—enhancing the value of personhood and more accurately perceiving self—are even more directly related to the material in this poem. For example, it seems likely that participants will come to consider attitudes and feelings about self (Objective 3) both because of the use of first-person pronouns and because of the reflective tone of the poem. The strong mood established by Frost also makes this a work likely to stimulate emotions, moods, and feelings (Objective 4). So, too, the images and refrain about "miles to go before I sleep" suggests future time as well as distance and might well lead to considerations of the process of time, growth, and change (Objective 5). The strong visual images in the poem might evoke memories for some participants (Objective 6). And, if the session concentrated on reflections about what various participants felt they should or shouldn't do because of "promises to keep," some groups might consider chemical dependency as it affects self (Objective 7). But it is unlikely that this poem will lead to considerations of the human body (Objectives 1 and 2).

The third goal, to recognize the reality and potentiality of interpersonal relationships, is the one least likely to become the focus of a dialogue stimulated by this poem. Not only does the imagery emphasize the speaker alone with his reflections, but there is little direct reference to interactions with others to begin with (the owner of the woods does not see the driver, for example). However, the idea of "promises to keep" might move some participants to exploring responsibilities they think they may have pledged to family or friends (Objectives 7 and 8) or to considering frustration or success in relationships that are related to the way the participant did or did not live up to expectations (Objective 4).

On the other hand, Frost's poem is very likely to be a catalyst for discussions built around the fourth goal—increasing reality-orientation. In particular, considerations of life-style and its meaning (Objective 2), life and its meaning (Objective 5), and death and its meaning (Objective 6) are natural foci for discussion.

Note that it is not enough simply to recognize that one of these objectives might be served by discussion of the poem. Indeed, it is also important to anticipate the precise direction of emphasis such a dialogue might take. For example, for some individuals the idea of a place dark and deep and remote from the pressures of dealing with others might seem to be a description of the attractions of suicide. Since suicide is one of the topics that must be handled with both skill and care, the facilitator should reconsider using this poem if the group includes a member who is likely to focus unproductively on the attractions of death as an escape.

However, deciding whether or not a particular work is *suitable* for use with a specific participant, group, or session is a somewhat different activity than evaluating whether or not a work has *potential* for use in bibliotherapy. The next chapter will look into the strategies the bibliotherapist uses to select material for a specific meeting of a specific group.

STUDY GUIDE

1. Concisely define the terms used in relation to thematic and stylistic dimensions in a way that would explain the criteria to someone unfamiliar with bibliotherapy. Indicate any criteria not included in the list that you personally feel are important.

2. Using insights gained from Allport (1937, 220–224), Arieti (1950), Cousins (1979), Moody (1978), or Plessner (1970), or from any other book or article on humor, draw up a statement on the value of humor in bibliotherapy. Choose three examples of humorous items that you consider usable with a specific group.

3. Write a statement that summarizes the relationship between the goals of bibliotherapy, the criteria used for evaluating bibliotherapeutic potential of materials, and the gauges.

4. Write your reaction to this statement (Turner 1980, 13): "The poem must speak to an individual *I* in order to reach the universal *I* and that individual *I* must originate in the poet; the individual *I* must not seem to be too private, too singular, lest it exclude the universal *I*." Then list one or two poems in which the *I* is so particularized that the universal is not apparent, and five in which the *I* is universalized.

PRACTICUM

1. Look for two poems you feel are lacking in strong potential for use in bibliotherapy and four that seem suitable. Use the thematic and stylistic dimensions given in this chapter to help you evaluate all six works. In a classroom situation, students of bibliotherapy should present and explain at least one of their choices and their ratings. (The authors would be interested in any serious alternate system of evaluating the bibliotherapeutic potential of material. Suggestions should be sent to them in care of Westview Press.)

2. Use the gauges to analyze at least two poems you consider suitable for bibliotherapy. If possible, use one of these poems either in a class experiential bibliotherapy group or with a group in which you are training. See if the points you noted in applying the gauges show up in the dialogue. Were there any directions taken that you did not anticipate?

FURTHER READINGS

Perrine (1962, 1969, 1978) offers clear, succinct discussions with examples of the standard features and devices found in poetry (1962, 1969) and in prose forms (1978). Perrine's texts are widely used for introductory college classes and constitute an invaluable resource for bibliotherapists who wish to brush up on their awareness of literary criteria. Jalongo (1983b) very briefly indicates the general criteria for selecting items for bibliotherapeutic use with children. See also Huck (1976), whose work is discussed in Chapter 6.

5

Strategic Choice of Bibliotherapeutic Materials

Let us look at the strategic decisions involved in choosing materials during a series of sessions for a bibliotherapy group of hospitalized drug addicts.

Early in January, members of this group read Lucille Clifton's poem "I'm Running into a New Year." The discussion revolved around the members' own struggles to build a new life. At the end of the meeting, the participants were asked to write personal responses to the title of the Clifton poem. Before the next meeting the facilitator typed copies of the original writings to enhance their use as the material for the next session.

Because the group was large, it took two meetings to read aloud and react to each person's poem. Members appreciated the concepts that thinking about walls and fences had "kicked up in them," as they put it. So, when the last of the original writings had been presented, they asked the bibliotherapist to find a poem that would keep them on the same subject the next time.

The facilitator first thought of Robert Frost's "Mending Walls." But most of the participants in this group had had little in the way of personal experience to bring to Frost's description of a rural scene.

Although a film version of Frost's poem might have bridged the experiential gap, this film had distracted an earlier group from the interpersonal issues in which the present participants had expressed an interest. In the end, the bibliotherapist provided copies of the text and read the poem aloud. The subsequent discussion of Frost's poem led some participants to explore how they had previously walled themselves into prisons of self.

As this dialogue implied themes of opening and closing, the facilitator chose the poem "Regarding a Door" by D. Antin for the next session. The poem might well have been too confusing for other clinical groups, but the bibliotherapist knew that most of the present group members were attentive and liked innovative material. She was confident that they would work through the poem verse by verse.

At the close of the session, the members wrote again on their feelings about the issues brought out by the discussion. It took another two meetings to go around the circle and dialogue about each member's writing.

At the close of these sessions, circumstances provided a totally new topic. A man who had graduated from the program three years before stopped by the hospital and sat in at the second meeting, during which the members' original writings were being discussed. In the course of relating how he had built a new life for himself, he strongly recommended one of the selections he remembered best from the bibliotherapy group. He then recited the lyrics for Cat Stevens's rather long song, "I'm on the Road to Find Out."

The facilitator followed through by opening the next session with a recorded version of the song. The group members responded enthusiastically. Many felt that the song was almost autobiographical and that they, too, had found that "the answer lies within."

The bibliotherapist wanted to build on the momentum leading toward self-perception. Thus, at the next session she brought in several copies of poetry books and a few high-school literature textbooks from which the participants could choose a poem that appealed to them.

In each of the next several weeks, two or three participants read and discussed their choices. Although the group itself did not stop, the activity brought to a close this particular cycle of choices centered on related themes.

THE STRATEGIC CHOICE OF MATERIAL for a particular group involves a series of considerations:

1. Are the interests of the group best served by having the choice of literature made by the facilitator or by the participants themselves, or are they best served through the use of creative writing?
2. What life circumstances should be taken into account when choosing a selection, and how well does the selection speak to these particular participants' readiness for self-understanding or therapy?
3. How receptive are these participants to the style, format, or mode of representation of the given piece of literature?

We will consider each of these points in turn.

Responsibility for Choice of Bibliotherapeutic Materials

The first decision to be made for each session is whether the material will be selected either by the bibliotherapist or by the participants, or whether creative writing will be used.

Material chosen by the bibliotherapist

In most clinical and many developmental groups, the bibliotherapist usually decides that the needs of the individual participants will be best served if the bibliotherapist personally selects the item to be used as the tool for a specific session. After all, the bibliotherapist has been trained to be attuned to the needs of the members and sensitive to individual areas of growth.

In addition, bibliotherapists generally have files of materials that meet specific needs. At the same time, they have both an intuitive and a critical sense for what works, based on many hours of experience. Moreover, supervision and systematic self-evaluation will have sharpened their critical skills.

Quite aside from the bibliotherapist's qualifications, however, certain factors make it difficult or undesirable to ask participants to select the literature. Many retarded, learning-disabled, and mentally ill patients will not be able to recognize their needs or know how or where to obtain suitable materials. Furthermore, many items may need to be adapted before they can be used with such groups. Developmental group members may prefer to have suggestions made, or they may have a limited sense of what can be used and where interesting materials are to be found.

Material chosen by participants

In virtually all bibliotherapy groups, including those made up of very ill clinical participants, the facilitator will generally decide that the members can benefit from spending one or two meetings dialoguing about material that they themselves have selected. In the first place, the members express themselves by their very choices: They show what pleases them, touches them, or disturbs them. At a deeper level, the participants' search for suitable or relevant material heightens their awareness of what it is they want to express or question and of how the message or concept is communicated by different media or genre. Finally, interpersonal relationships can be strengthened by having group members choose the material. In this way, participants are given the chance to enjoy and share what they have found meaningful. As a result, some individuals will become aware both of problem areas and of strengths that they share with others. At the same time, the members will learn to assume responsibility for a group activity; some will become aware enough of others to look consciously for a piece that might be meaningful to other participants as well as to themselves.

As we will note again in the context of group dynamics (Chapter 12), participants are sometimes more receptive to a poem chosen by another group member and may be willing to discuss issues that they would resist if the initiative came from the facilitator. For example, one member of a clinical group brought in Nikki Giovanni's "Legacies." The initial response of the other participants was mixed. But when a young woman said, "We don't say what we mean to others—I don't say what I mean easily," more than one member looked at her carefully and then looked away or shifted positions. The facilitator had previously tried—unsuccessfully—to get the participants to discuss what they personally felt about communicating with others; but now they tentatively began to explore how likely they were to say what they meant. The remark triggered by a participant's choice of material finally brought about some dialogue on the issue.

We will detail the procedures involved in facilitating the actual selection process in Chapter 9.

Creative writing

Bibliotherapists should recognize that there are times when the participants will benefit from engaging in the special kind of thought and reflection that comes from making a response in writing rather than voicing it as part of a discussion. If nothing else, writing involves every member of the group in an externalized response. However, there is no rule of thumb about who will respond well when the activity is actually initiated. Some participants who would never say that they wanted to write can produce very useful material; others who have trouble expressing themselves orally may find release in writing. Yet at different times in the course of a bibliotherapy group, the same individual may be blocked at one point and able to write with ease at another.

Participants who are fearful of or unaccustomed to writing should be eased into using this mode of expression. Furthermore, creative writing should not be used until the group climate is characterized by cohesiveness and mutual concern. Otherwise, participants may show signs of boredom, inattention, or hostility when others' selections are being discussed.

Note that the degree to which creative writing is used as material is a question of personal style. Some bibliotherapists often have group members write; in fact, some feel it is the most productive source of material. Others, however, do not find it as easy to initiate or facilitate discussions based on the participant's own writings; still others feel that exposure to literature stimulates responses that self-expression will not bring out. All of these positions are legitimate. The important thing is that the bibliotherapist must be personally comfortable with the approach that is being used.

More often than not, the strategy for choosing material is arrived at in a way similar to that indicated in the opening case study: The facilitator considers the three options and plans each session as the circumstances warrant.

Influence of Participants' Life Circumstances on Choice of Bibliotherapeutic Materials

Because the bibliotherapeutic material is meant to act as a catalyst, it is critical that the chosen item have some inherent appeal and relevance to the members. The age and educational level, the physical and mental health, and the specific living conditions of the participants (e.g., prison, hospice, support group, etc.) all influence the choice of material for a given session with a given group or individual.

We will briefly look in turn at the special considerations and/or resources that the bibliotherapist should be aware of with respect to each of these factors.

Age and educational level

Children and adolescents. A superabundance of material exists that can be used bibliotherapeutically with children and adolescents. In addition to juvenile publications, the bibliotherapist can refer to many annotated lists of titles dealing with the kinds of problems faced by children and adolescents. For example, both Cacha (1978) and Watson (1980) have selected materials appropriate for use with abused children. Bowker (1982) and Martin et al. (1983) list books for children coping with divorce, whereas Rossi (1983) has compiled a list of twenty-eight picture books that feature single-parent families and Wallick (1980) discusses books pertaining to autistic children. Among the bibliographies that include listings for more than one problem are Berg-Cross and Berg-Cross (1976), Bracken and Wigotoff (1979), Jalongo (1983a), Overstad (1981), and Thomas and Vaughan (1983). In addition, Compton and Skelton (1982) have analyzed fifteen of the most currently popular adolescent novels to see what social problems these books are dealing with.

Note that some of these lists understand bibliotherapy to be a reading process rather than an interactive one. Many of the resources listed at the end of Chapter 6 also contain many useful items but do not mention bibliotherapy as such. In the end, then, the vast range of literature available suggests that the facilitator must be very discriminating in deciding what specific item will actually be effective with a given child or group at a specific time.

Those who work with children soon discover that they must be very sensitive not just to the themes in a work but also to the way the participants are likely to react to the style and presentation of the material. Children are particularly resistant to examining anything that they feel is "boring." The bibliotherapist will have to determine whether "boring" either masks avoidance or indicates that the items look too serious or too dull. Although the presentation should not detract from the emphasis on response, the bibliotherapist can sometimes overcome resistance by using complementary materials or presenting the material in a lively or unexpected way.

Students, too, can be very conservative about what they think is appropriate. For example, song lyrics can be a powerful tool, but some devotees of popular music may resent any attempt to make their entertainment "meaningful."

By the same token, some children will withdraw from literature that forces them into direct confrontation with a troublesome issue. Thus children trying to cope with the breakup of their family may strongly resist making any personal applications from a story that is actually about children and divorce.

Poor readers. Reading level can have a significant impact on the effectiveness of a particular item. In addition to young children, learning-disabled people, retarded individuals, prisoners, chemically addicted persons, and chronically ill mental patients may be barely literate and thus may find the process of getting through the material so laborious, frustrating, or humiliating that they have no impetus to make a feeling-response.

Poor readers of adult age are often very sensitive about their problem and may resist using anything that looks "like a kid's book." One effective solution is oral presentation; in other cases the bibliotherapist may wish to adapt and/or retype the material. Possible adjustments include substituting easier words, shortening sentences, or typing each passage in short phrase units. Poetry, on the other hand, is by nature such an economical form that it generally cannot be adapted in this way. If one poem causes difficulty, the bibliotherapist would do better to look for another in which the vocabulary and syntax are simpler.

Aging individuals. In a sense, almost anything is adaptable for use with aging people. But different issues will be important to different groups. Some members will be most concerned with trying to adjust to and find meaning in a daily life that is very different from the one they led as working people. Others will be focused on life review. Elderly chronic patients can be so lethargic and withdrawn that even the most basic kind of stimulation or interaction would amount to a significant success in treatment.

The analysis by Sohngen and Smith (1978) of the treatment of aging individuals in the poems listed in *Granger's Index to Poetry* is an excellent lesson in how lists of references like this should be used critically. The analysis shows that many poems designated as dealing with the theme of age are actually about something else; furthermore, many of the 127 poems that Sohngen and Smith see as truly based on this theme are fundamentally negative about aging and thus are unsuitable for bibliotherapy.

Although he does not treat bibliotherapy directly, McLeish (1976) sees growth as a continuous process; he raises many issues that the bibliotherapist must be sensitive to when choosing material or inviting creative writing from senior citizens. L. Allen (1981) and Koch (1977) do not see themselves as bibliotherapists, but both have developed effective techniques that can be adapted for encouraging creative writing with elderly persons.

Some of the articles about bibliotherapy with aging individuals cited in Chapter 1 identify specific materials that have been used successfully. Additional resources are listed in Chapter 6. Although these latter items were not designed specifically for bibliotherapy, they have proven valuable.

Mental and physical condition

Mental patients. Bibliotherapists choosing materials for mentally ill patients will have to take into account needs specific to different types and degrees of mental illness. For example, people diagnosed as manic and other agitated patients often have a very short attention span. The facilitator might find it necessary to have several related items in reserve for introduction in the course of a single session. Or, as earlier noted, chronic patients may need a great deal of stimulus to become more aware of the world around them; the facilitator in that case would rely heavily on short, very concrete poems that can be reinforced with complementary materials. On the other hand, some patients are not able to focus when presented with intense stimuli such as those found in films.

The bibliotherapist in a mental-health setting often works as part of a treatment team, keeping records as well as consulting with other staff members about the participants. Those who do not have a background in mental-health work should look for readings and supervision that will make them more aware of both general and individual patterns of behavior and response that are symptomatic of illness. It is particularly important to avoid material that would in some way feed an individual's schizoid fantasizing or suicidal tendencies.

Blind persons. Most of the limitations with respect to materials that can be used effectively with blind participants do not really reflect thematic concerns. But special consideration should be given to how readily the ideas or images can be grasped if the text is only heard and not seen. It makes sense, as well, to seek out items that appeal more to the senses of sound, touch, taste, or smell—senses that the blind do have—rather than to use works with strongly visual images. Some bibliotherapists look for complementary material (such as the jingle bells used with hospitalized blind mental patients) to increase the impact of the text.

Braille books, talking books, and other cassette materials are especially valuable for the blind. In addition, the bibliotherapist can consult the local public library or service for the blind as well as the National Library Service for the Blind and Physically Handicapped (Library of Congress, Washington, DC 20542).

Deaf persons. Any bibliotherapist working with deaf participants will need to be familiar with the pertinent methods of communication, including lip-reading, the manual alphabet, and the American Sign Language (ASL). If the facilitator is not personally fluent in the mode used by a given group, he or she should arrange for an interpreter. In addition, the facilitator must ensure that all members can easily see each other's signing or lip-reading. Note, too, that as the signing of descriptive words is particularly difficult, poems that rely heavily on adjectives or contain many metaphors and abstractions may lose their effectiveness when interpreted into sign language.

Batson and Berfman (1976) do not specifically mention bibliotherapy, but the readings in their book will alert facilitators to deaf participants' special needs and interests.

Individuals with other disabilities. Bibliotherapists can consult with a speech therapist about techniques to use in dialoguing with stroke victims or others whose speech has been affected. Freytag (1977) suggests some materials and techniques specifically designed for bibliotherapy with speech-impaired children.

Regarding subject matter, the bibliotherapist can refer to certain bibliographies of stories and poems that deal with handicaps (e.g., Greenbaum et al. 1980; Huck 1976, 426–435; Marshall 1981). They might also look for items concerned with more generalized themes such as persistence, frustration, dealing with limitations, or self-perception. In addition, didactic health education materials can help correct misunderstandings about the disability and can provide an opportunity for venting feelings.

Life condition

The choice of bibliotherapeutic material is also influenced by needs the members share because of a given life situation.

Prisoners. Many sessions for prisoners develop around works that explore the need for mutual respect for others and for authority or that help the participants find ways to express anger and frustration appropriately. However, as there seems to be strong connection between crime and poor academic performance, facilitators for prisoner groups should familiarize themselves with and draw on all the easy reading materials available for adults.

At the same time, the facilitator should try to use items that reflect and can be found in the world from which the participants come. For instance, *Ebony, Life, People,* and *Essence* feature articles, poems, and photographic stories, but—equally important—they are sources that the participants can easily find and return to on their own. On occasion, the bibliotherapist may also extract passages from such "prison literature" as Eldridge Cleaver's *Soul on Ice* or *The Autobiography of Malcolm X.*

Even when the material deals with some relevant specific factual matter, the focus should still be bibliotherapeutic. A bibliotherapist might bring in a job application to be filled out, for instance. Some time would undoubtedly be spent in clarifying what specific kind of information is being requested and what kinds of records participants should expect to have on hand. But the bibliotherapist should also use the dialogue to help the participants face and cope with the shame some feel at having to acknowledge their prison record, or the anger and frustration that others experience because they find the mechanics of filling out the form so difficult.

Drug and alcohol groups. Short-term programs are designed to intensively help members recognize and then overcome their dependencies. The material for such groups will usually deal quite directly with these issues. A movie like *Days of Wine and Roses* or an old poem like "The Face on the Barroom Floor" provides significant opportunity for reaction. Alan Dungan's "Prayer" and Paul L. Dunbar's "The Debt" speak of the bitter aftermath of addiction. The bibliotherapist might also refer to Alcoholics Anonymous for good sources of material; in particular, Swift (1983) argues for the therapeutic value of *The Blue Book* and the *Twelve Steps and Twelve Traditions* in recovery programs.

It is not necessary that all of the literature mention addiction directly. As we saw in the opening vignette, issues of self-imprisonment, of the need to love and depend more on oneself, and of the need to recognize one's limits can be reflected in many different images. In addition, some bibliotherapeutic programs have successfully devoted several months to a chapter-by-chapter discussion of certain nonfiction books such as Eric Berne's *Games People Play* or Erich Fromm's *The Art of Loving.*

Bibliotherapy participants in long-term addiction programs may want to use the selected literature to develop broader interests. In this connection, one group of women in a year-long program asked the bibliotherapist to provide them with other topics of conversational and recreational usefulness. They said that in the process of moving beyond the desperate stage, they began to recognize that their social drinking had begun at an early age because they had so few interests and so little confidence in their ability to be interested or interesting. By contrast, the materials the bibliotherapist had used in the past months had opened up all kinds of topics to talk about. As a consequence, the participants felt that the bibliotherapy was challenging them to become whole persons. They mentioned how both their self-esteem and their horizons had been extended through the new insights they had acquired from the lyrics of familiar songs or through their introduction to ethnic literature.

Hospice programs. Bibliotherapists working with dying individuals will have to be extremely sensitive to their needs and capabilities. The degree to which material should directly address the critical issues and feelings connected with death and dying will vary from one person to another and will change during the course of the illness.

Whether or not the following works are used in a particular session, the facilitator should be familiar with Elizabeth Kubler-Ross's (1969, 1975, 1978) work on the six stages of denial, isolation, anger, bargaining, depression, and acceptance. Ewens and Harrington's (1982) chapter on "Grief as Growth" and Moody's (1964) article provide valuable discussions of the grieving process. Although it would often be inappropriate to use these works with the patient personally, the families may find this kind of material very helpful in dealing with the painful process of separation and grief. Kobak (1975), for instance, points to certain techniques she has found helpful in working with widows.

Since the patient is often exhausted by illness, both the material and the dialogue may have to be quite short. Poetry, given its economy and evocativeness, is an especially powerful genre.

Support groups. Facilitators of developmental bibliotherapy groups formed around a common interest are likely to turn to material that has been identified on the basis of a given theme or situation. Such material might comprise, for instance, the lists and anthologies of works for and about women and their status and problems. Certainly these resources are a good place to start. But once again, it is not enough for an item to be *about* a given theme; style and treatment must also be evaluated in terms of the overall criteria used to gauge the effectiveness of the material in question.

However, as valuable as specialized bibliographies can be when used with discrimination, the literature intended for specific groups should never be limited to items that deal explicitly with the relevant issue or situation. There is no indication in Mari Evans's "The Silver Cell" of the speaker's sex or life circumstances, for example. But this short poem's assertion that the speaker is personally responsible for his (or her) own prison, and is both slave and master, has been a very powerful tool for dialogue in women's groups as well as in groups of participants struggling with chemical dependency.

Physical environment. Although a good choice of material with nature imagery is available, the bibliotherapist may have difficulty finding good urban poetry in which the images are universally applicable to daily life. The following three sources may be your best bet: Nancy Larrick's *On City*

Streets and A. Adoff's anthology *City in All Directions* present many aspects of city life; Langston Hughes's *The Best of Simple* depicts a black man who meets the difficult situations in his urban environment with humor and wisdom.

Even though participants may not have much experience with nature, bibliotherapists should not automatically rule out works that use nature imagery. In fact, we see here another aspect of the principle that the choice of material should not be too restrictive. The facilitator can purposely select items that increase the participants' capacity to respond more fully to the realities of their world. The sky, the lone tree or bush, the nearby park, flowers in a window box, the rain, the fog, and the snow are all features of the world of nature that are present virtually everywhere.

At the same time, a renewed awareness of the physical world will increase the impact and accessibility of poems that use images from nature to make powerful statements about daily life. For example, Frost's poem "Lodged" begins with the rain talking to the wind about pushing and pelting the flowers, and ends with: "I know how the flowers felt." All of us have felt the wind and rain, and all of us have been pushed and pelted by forces in our lives. Discussion of this poem along with nature photographs of rainfall or of plants and trees beaten by the wind, or accompanied by a recording of a rainstorm can bring the poem to life even for those who live in a denatured environment. Such sensitive, strategic choices about presentation can help prisoners, addicts, mental patients, and those with physical problems use the poem to talk about the feelings they often have about having lost control of their lives. Moreover, children may begin to vent feelings about the way they see adults, and elderly parents can make a connection with the way they feel manipulated by their children.

Materials that reflect the history of the group

It may seem that this discussion of how to choose materials that address specific factors such as age or life situations is not terribly detailed. But, in fact, there is a limit to how precise any such guidelines can be. In the end, it is not enough for the facilitator to identify overall needs and interests; he or she must be aware of the way that individuals in a given group translate these needs and conditions into specific feelings and issues. The mix that must be taken into account is inevitably unique for each group and each individual member.

But we have already suggested another reason that bibliotherapists cannot possibly draw up anything as precise as a syllabus or even establish a file that is sure to contain material for a given group. As we saw in the opening vignette, the facilitator chooses material for any given session in light of what has taken place in previous meetings. In other words, the facilitator draws on the specific *experiences of the group* as well as on his or her overall experience in bibliotherapy. In Chapter 12 we will discuss in more detail the ways in which a facilitator can adapt strategies and materials to various points in the life span of a group.

Strategies Pertaining to Genre and Media

In addition to considering life circumstances, the bibliotherapist must determine which genre or media is best suited to stimulate dialogue with a particular group at a particular time.

Poetry

Poetry is often the best tool with which to provide an ordered and condensed presentation of an experience to the broadest range of individuals. Not only are poems usually of a suitable length, but their images and metaphors tend to appeal simultaneously to the senses, emotions, and intelligence as well as to the imagination. Good poetry is precise and, at the same time, can elicit responses on many different levels. Thus some participants will respond to the message and beauty on a literal level, while others in the same group will very quickly move on to the symbolic meaning and to an integration of the insights into their personal lives.

We have already discussed themes, such as nature, that are common to lyric poetry. Insufficient space limits our discussion of different poetic forms, but suffice to note that song lyrics are poetry and can be very effective tools in bibliotherapy. The words of ballads, folk songs, spirituals, and popular music (including rock and country tunes) tend to reflect themes about human emotions as well as to use effectively such stylistic techniques as rhythm, repetition, and rhyme. Participants may associate a song with someone else or with some experience. Those who do not know the song can find release in the aesthetic impact of words and music, and may even come to some recognition because of the phrasing. Of course, the bibliotherapist may also decide to present the lyrics alone, without referring to the music, as in some cases resistance to the style of music or preoccupation with the performance in a recording can distract members from the meaning of the lyrics.

Not all persons respond immediately to poetry, however. The bibliotherapist may have to begin by relying more on another genre until the suspicion or prejudice against poetry breaks down. At other times the facilitator will not be able to find a suitable poem for the issues he or she feels the group needs to address. But there are situations in which poetry is not a good choice of genre to begin with. As indicated in the earlier discussion of criteria, participants who are very literal may have trouble with the symbolic level of many poems. In other cases, the very powerful potential of poetry will prompt the bibliotherapist to decide against it—particularly in a mental hospital or prison, where the atmosphere or issue may be too charged to use poetry. In that case, the more relaxed approach of a short story, article, or film might be better for bringing the issue to dialogue.

Imaginative prose

Short stories, fables, science fiction, fantasy tales, novels, and plays are all forms of imaginative prose that can be used or adapted for use in bibliotherapy. With experience, the bibliotherapist will become better aware of the advantages and contra-indications for each. But, again, as we indicated in the discussion of criteria, length can be a significant issue. In dealing with prose forms, the bibliotherapist generally must either extract a passage that will be meaningful on its own or make some arrangement for having the reading done ahead of time.

In addition, story line and character are central elements in most imaginative prose. When deciding on the therapeutic potential of a particular work, the bibliotherapist should consider criteria such as those proposed by Lundsteen (1964) and adapted by Kanaan (1975) to bibliotherapy. A story that includes the features indicated by the following questions would be a strong candidate for use:

1. Are significant relevant problems dealt with?
2. Are the characters believable?
3. Are enough conditions given that the reader can either analyze the parts of the problem to be dealt with or use the depicted situation to create a hypothesis that might help the character in situations involving significant human relationships?
4. Do the participants gain something by sharing this literature?
5. Can an unfinished episode from the book be extracted so that the participants can propose their own alternative ways to deal with the problem or situation?

Informational material

In addition to imaginative works, bibliotherapists can use various forms of nonfiction prose to help participants clarify their personal reactions to the ways in which facts or theories impinge on their lives. In general, the language of nonfiction is meant to involve the intellect rather than to re-create an experience—even though the rhetoric of nonfiction does frequently include a definite emotional, persuasive element.

Sketches and articles. These forms tend to be short and often use writing that is lively and meant to catch the reader's interest from the start. Both can be found in the feature pages of newspapers, in magazines, and in collections of essays. Apathetic persons, learning-disabled or retarded individuals, and very emotionally disturbed patients who are not used to the bibliotherapeutic approach can begin to find their interest stimulated by the readily grasped writing characteristic of many sketches and articles. We will note later how these forms can be used to introduce or close a session in which other material has been used.

Not all essays or sketches should be considered as fillers. We have cited several examples in which biographical sketches offered models that participants used to examine their own actions and attitudes. Feature stories or short newspaper columns, too, may vividly capture situations or feelings from daily life in a way that stimulates a good discussion.

However, the bibliotherapist will find it unproductive to use items such as current events stories detailing disasters or events that have strong emotional impact but offer little personal meaning for the participants other than a reinforcement of feelings of fear, helplessness, or despair. The point of effective bibliotherapy is not to stir emotions but to integrate them.

Factual information. Factual information about physical or mental health, or about skills or issues that have a direct impact on the participant's life, is also potentially useful in bibliotherapy. In this case, the objective is to help the individual recognize and work out his or her *emotional* response to the nature and consequences of the disease as well as to the need for a particular treatment. For example, we feel that bibliotherapy would be a valuable component in hospital *patient education* programs in which factual information about disease and its control is provided. Diabetic, asthmatic, manic-depressive, and other patients whose well-being depends on taking medicine regularly may find bibliotherapy an effective way to talk out the messages to self that might be masked in carelessness or resistance to medication.

When working with the educational staff of a hospital or correctional institution, the bibliotherapist should either use the didactic material directly in a bibliotherapeutic way or bring in complementary bibliotherapeutic materials as an immediate follow-up to a teaching session. As a last resort, the facilitator could use the informational material in both an educational and a therapeutic way.

Rational-emotive therapists also advocate the use of didactic material. Although such therapists tend to identify bibliotherapy with reading, the therapy itself does rely on many interactive techniques (Ellis 1969; Roberts 1982; Maultsby 1984). Thus there is no fundamental incompatibility between the two approaches. In fact, bibliotherapists might use the rational-emotive approach as a model for expanding the use of didactic materials. The mix of imaginative and didactic passages can be very effective. For example, bibliotherapy growth/self-improvement groups sponsored by an employer might use one of the self-help manuals recommended by Glasgow and Rosen (1978) in their evaluative survey.

Audiovisual materials

Although written texts can be used in virtually any bibliotherapy session, there are certain technical restrictions as to when and where audiovisuals can be employed. In addition, the extent to which audiovisuals are used tends to reflect the personal style of the bibliotherapist. In any case, our experience has shown that printed and audiovisual materials are absorbed and responded to in different ways and to varying degrees; indeed, we hope that further research will explore more thoroughly the nature of these differences in bibliotherapeutic impact.

Elias (1983) has done some very interesting work with disturbed adolescents using videotaped television shows. Kilguss's (1974) analysis of the portrayal of women in soap operas is no longer valid; even so, she makes some very thought-provoking observations about how and why soap operas can provide a very stimulating focus for therapeutic dialogue.

Commercials are another important reflection of cultural expectations and assumptions, and, as such, may be of use to a skillful facilitator. For example, a bibliotherapy group for chemically dependent patients could look at video recordings of the popular beer commercials and examine the ways in which they reflect or distort the participants' actual experience or attitudes when drinking.

Conclusion

The strategic choice of materials for a particular bibliotherapy session involves a juggling of many factors, including consideration of the participants' life circumstances, choice of mode, and recognition of the impact of different genre. But a great deal depends on the facilitator's ability to make the right choice: The effectiveness of the tool—the chosen literature—often dictates how effective the bibliotherapeutic encounter will be. Clearly the bibliotherapist should expect to spend a significant amount of time selecting the literature. In the next chapter, we will outline some of the procedures and sources that can make this task easier.

STUDY GUIDE

1. Summarize the strategic considerations you must weigh as a bibliotherapist in deciding who should be responsible for the material at a given session. Include some specific advantages for the three alternatives: selection of material by the facilitator, selection by participants, and use of creative writing.

2. Compare and contrast the different factors and life-interests that would have to be taken into account when choosing material for two different populations.

3. Identify the characteristic differences in content-emphasis, in treatment, and in appeal for each of the three major categories of material: imaginative writings, nonfiction prose, and audiovisuals. Indicate the category you would personally feel most comfortable using. Try to analyze why you feel as you do and what implications your preference has for your practice of bibliotherapy.

PRACTICUM

1. Imagine yourself as a participant in a specific bibliotherapeutic group. Identify and characterize your needs. Then select three items that a bibliotherapist might choose to use in this situation. Explain how your choices reflect the overall criteria, your specific needs, and the strengths of the genre used.

2. Alternatively, review the literature about working with a specific population in which you are interested. Compile a list of all the works cited as having been used effectively in this context as bibliotherapeutic material. Locate as many items as you can to see if you can identify any patterns in the style, thematic focus, and treatment.

3. Find at least one item from each of the three general categories of material (imaginative literature, nonfiction prose, audiovisuals) that treats the same theme (e.g., separation, loneliness, hope, relationships between men and women). Then indicate the ways in which that genre or medium affects the treatment and potential impact of the theme. Finally, list the groups or circumstances in which you feel use of the piece would be either indicated or contra-indicated.

4. Read and report on at least one of the following discussions of the importance of story to self-understanding: Applebee (1978), Bettleheim (1976), Cox (1969), Crosson (1975), Fromm (1951), McConnell (1979), Singer (1973, 1975a), Tolkien (1974), Vanderpost (1972), Wilson (1979). In your report, define as precisely as possible how the author understands "story." For example does the term seem to designate any narrative, written or oral? Is the emphasis on fantasy, folklore, or day-dreaming? Is the analysis more concerned with the dynamics of telling or with those of listening? Then discuss how your own understanding of the material in the selection can be applied to bibliotherapy.

FURTHER READINGS

Refer to Pearle et al. (1982) for the U.S. government report on the studies that formed the basis for the Surgeon General's report entitled *Television and Behavior.* Anyone interested in exploring video-recorded selections from television as bibliotherapy material should familiarize themselves with this kind of research. Note that the studies are not confined to the impact of television on children.

Kaplan and Bean (1976), Kravetz and Jones (1981), and Tyler (1978) offer stimulating explorations of the concept of androgyny and its relationship to mental health. In reflecting on these studies you may clarify your emphasis on not restricting materials to those that are explicitly associated with the life circumstances of a given population.

6

Resources and the Management of Bibliotherapeutic Materials

As a clinical bibliotherapist looked for a poem on loneliness to use with a group of severely depressed patients, he reflected that each search for material is unique. Sometimes he was able to pull the perfect piece for the next meeting of a group out of the files immediately and almost effortlessly.

At other times, like today, nothing at hand seemed suitable. He had looked through all the items listed in his subject file under "loneliness" and "multifaceted." He had reluctantly passed by several possibilities. For example, the line in e.e. cummings's "maggie and milly and molly and may" that described may's stone as being "as small as a world and as large as alone" captured the tone he was looking for, but the main focus of the poem was really self-perception—a significant issue but not the one this group was ready for.

He now was paging through the collections and anthologies he kept on hand. If nothing seemed right, he would have to check for other leads in the library's resource materials.

The search really was unpredictable, he thought. The cummings poem would have been perfect for a session last month with the dependency program group. Now the short short story he was skimming looked very promising—but in another situation. He did pause long enough to make a copy so that he could add the work to his files. He knew that as the files grew and as experience built up, the likelihood that he'd find something useful on hand would become greater and greater.

After several hours of intensive searching, the bibliotherapist finally came across a poem in a recent magazine. He was relieved; but even so, as demanding as it was, he did not find the search for the right material to be frustrating. Rather, he regarded refining and honing the files as part of the creative challenge of bibliotherapy.

Sources for Bibliotherapeutic Materials

ON ONE LEVEL, BIBLIOTHERAPISTS regard everything they read as potential material. Every time they glance through the newspaper, scan magazines at home or in the library, browse in a second-hand bookstore or in a music store, or check through the film and record sections at local libraries, they are alert for items to add to the files. More times than not, the search—either for something to use with a specific group or to build up the files—is quite deliberate.

In this chapter, we will indicate the resources to consult and the procedures to follow when filing and indexing materials. The chapter ends with a selected bibliography of useful reference books.

Lists, anthologies, and collections

Every bibliotherapist will have his or her own method of searching and will develop sources that are likely to yield effective materials.

1. Those working with handicapped individuals, with regressed chronic mental patients, or with participants who are uncomfortable with highly symbolic material find anthologies of poetry for young people, such as those by Nancy Larrick, to be quite valuable. For the most part, such selections use commonplace vocabulary, universal subject matter, and concrete imagery that allow them to appeal to a wide range of participants.

2. Many bibliotherapists also scan general reading lists for children and adolescents for materials that might be useful. Although some items are unmistakably juvenile, others treat universal themes while still others can be adapted for use with adults. Lists that include the reading level for many works are helpful for those facilitators working with adult poor readers.

3. Although bibliographies of general interest materials for adults are less common, facilitators might want to examine critically the works listed or anthologized for specific groups. Many collections are designed to reflect ethnic interests, for instance. The following should give the reader some idea of what is available: Adoff (1973) and S. Allen (1973) both include poems that reflect the black experience; T. Allen (1972) has gathered poems about and by American Indians; and one might even refer to the *Anthology of Armenian Poetry*, edited by Der Hovanessian and Morgassian (1978). This last book in particular is a good example of how works that have been

collected under one heading can be relevant to all kinds of participants. In the same way, many Hassidic tales provide short, pithy statements about human needs and experiences in general.

4. High-school or college literature textbooks are good sources of a wide range of poems, short stories, and essays that relate to common experiences and basic themes such as using one's talents well, sibling relationships, making friends, overcoming handicaps, coming to terms with authority, and so on. People of every age and condition can also relate to the emotions of love and hate, fear, anger, joy, compassion, and sorrow that are touched on in many of these selections.

5. In addition, the bibliotherapist can refer to any of the innumerable *poetry anthologies* in existence. Some, such as those compiled by Perrine (1962, 1969, 1978), are designed for classroom use.

6. And, finally, there are those writers whose poems seem to have been designed specifically for bibliotherapeutic use. The present authors turn regularly to our editions of the collected works of Robert Frost, Langston Hughes, and Carl Sandburg, for example. We have also acquired collections of several less-known poets, such as Laura Gilpin, Valerie Worth, and Eve Merriam, whose works are equally rich resources.

Bibliotherapists' lists

Trainees who are still working on building files and developing their intuitions about what materials have strong potential as bibliotherapeutic tools will be especially interested in consulting bibliographies compiled by biblio/poetry therapists. In the previous chapter we cited a number of articles that contain such lists. In addition, J. J. Leedy's first book includes the titles of the materials he had used (1969, 276–280). The poems, plays, and short stories that Clara Lack had used in California are listed in *Using Bibliotherapy* (edited by Rubin, 1978a, 173–199). The same volume also includes Rubin's "Suggested Juvenile Materials for Bibliotherapy" (pp. 119–172).

Two reading specialists who use bibliotherapy very specifically as part of the reading process have also published bibliographies. Jacquelyn Stephens (1981, 36–39) lists items by subject areas, and Schultheis (1972), of the Institute for the Study of Bibliotherapy, Inc., not only includes a bibliography in her book but also periodically provides an annotated update of books designed to build a child's self-esteem (see *News and Reviews*, which is published eight times a year). The Bibliotherapy Discussion Group Newsletter, published by the American Library Association, also frequently describes professional literature of value as references for bibliotherapists and, less often, lists specific titles for use in bibliotherapy.

As the field of bibliotherapy grows, more lists and even anthologies of promising items are likely to appear.

General resources

Bibliotherapists-in-training are well-advised to take library-school courses in reference materials and book-selection techniques. Library schools and education departments also offer courses in children's or young adult's literature that provide a useful introduction to specific titles and resources in the field. For example, Huck (1976) lists hundreds of items after each chapter, often with some brief evaluation or notation in her text. She does not discuss bibliotherapy as such, but she does present and explain criteria for selecting material in a thoughtful way. At the same time, many of the poems she quotes in full in the eighty pages devoted to poetry have high potential as material to be used with adult as well as with juvenile bibliotherapy participants. Arbuthnot and Sutherland (1976) also offer a good textbook in this field.

By the same token, classes in the literature of various cultures or poetry, short story, or film classes can help broaden the bibliotherapist's familiarity with the literature available. Note that even though the instructor's emphasis is likely to be on aesthetic values, the bibliotherapist would look at how different items could improve self-understanding.

In a way, libraries and librarians are naturals for bibliotherapy. Each library is a storehouse of books and, in many communities, of audiovisual materials, but it also provides many useful reference tools for locating materials; librarians, of course, are trained to be skilled users of these resources.

A selected reference list for locating bibliotherapeutic materials is located at the end of the chapter. By no means exhaustive, this list should nonetheless indicate what kind of bibliographic and other reference tools are available. This list includes general resources, poetry indexes, lists of poetry, short stories, fairy tales, folklore, fantasy tales, science fiction, plays, materials designated for children and youth, films and other audiovisual materials, records, and multisensory media. Few periodicals are included, but facilitators should regularly scan magazines that feature fiction, poetry, and short articles. The local librarian can assist patrons in locating and using the reference tools on hand.

Identification of Bibliotherapeutic Materials

Items that have been located and selected as bibliotherapeutic materials should be both filed and indexed. We will look in turn at the procedures for storing and for indexing written materials, complementary materials, and audiovisuals.

Files of written texts

Both the master and the duplicate files of written bibliotherapeutic materials should be stored safely in a file cabinet readily accessible to the bibliotherapists who will use them in the process of selecting literature for use in a given session. We strongly recommend including single-sheet typescripts or copies of all items in these files. Even when the volume from which a printed selection was taken is at hand, it is much easier to scan items from an indexed file. As we have seen, such scanning is a regular feature of the bibliotherapist's routine—even for those with good recall. Particularly in larger institutions, such as mental hospitals, it is important to have the material both filed and indexed, as more than one person may be consulting and adding to the files.

Master files. The master file for written materials should include single copies of poems, plays, songs, short stories, articles, and excerpts. Items should be neatly typed or photocopied on standard-sized sheets of paper; in general, use double-spacing and one side only.

We also recommend the following format for including information on the master file copy:

- File all items alphabetically by author, with multiple selections from one author interfiled by title. Type the author's name, last name first, in the upper left-hand corner of each sheet of paper.
- Put the title of the material in quotation marks in the upper right-hand corner, about one inch down.
- Center the material on the page, and maintain a margin of an inch to an inch and a half all the way around.
- At the bottom margin, include both the title of the book from which the selection was taken and the publication information.
- On a separate line, indicate the pages on which the material appeared.

In general, the bibliotherapist should immediately return the materials to the master file after use, especially if the files are used by more than one person.

Duplicate files. Copies of materials to be distributed to participants can be stored in a duplicate file. When there is only one user, the duplicates may be filed with the originals. When copies of a particular item are almost depleted, make a note on a card kept at the front of the file so that several selections can be duplicated at once. Since mimeographed and carbon copies often smudge and tend to be hard to read, photocopies should be used whenever possible.

We cannot stress enough the importance of providing attractive, readable copies of the material for each participant. Sharp, clean, well-spaced copy is inviting; poorly typed, crowded, or smudged texts create a barrier between the reader and the text.

More important, some participants may even consciously or unconsciously read a message about the facilitator's respect for the material and/or the participants into the care with which the material is presented.

If you are using a typescript from the master file, block out the bibliographic information before photocopying duplicates for participants; the spontaneous response of some participants may actually be disrupted by the sight of the author's name.

If the master file entry is a photocopy of the pages of a book or magazine, you may find it worthwhile to retype the material in a different format for presentation to the bibliotherapy participants. For example, many people find it easier to follow short articles, stories, and poetry that have been centered on the page, double-spaced, and typed on special large-face machines. (If such a machine is not available, use all capital letters.) Particularly those participants who have any kind of reading problem will find it easier to follow large print.

In addition, clearly mark the space between paragraphs or stanzas with three or four empty lines. You can also adapt prose texts by typing the paragraphs into segments that represent complete thoughts. Not only weak readers will find it easier to master the material, but also those who are overly absorbed in their own problems will be better able to focus on the content of each small segment of a selection in order to follow the discussion. Furthermore, generous spacing makes it easier to find a passage in referring back to the text.

According to the relevant points of the copyright law (U.S. Congress 1970), there are no restrictions on duplicating materials that are in the public domain; hence you can make copies of poems, stories, songs, and essays that were published more than seventy years ago. It is also legal to copy any writing that does not have a copyright. In addition, the law allows you to make one reproduction of copyrighted material without asking permission from the publisher. In short, there is no restriction to building up your master file.

At the same time, the copyright law on fair use (Item 10) allows copies of an item that is being used as the basis for comment, as in a classroom. However, it expressly forbids the collection of a series of copyrighted material into a booklet—even if there is no question of selling involved. Technically, any such collection is considered by the law to be an anthology.

On the other hand, some libraries or other institutions may have acquired multiple copies of textbooks or anthologies that can be used for participant-selected material. There are no restrictions on using such anthologies, of course. The facilitator will usually decide to collect and store the books between sessions so that they cannot be lost or forgotten by participants.

Shelved files. In addition to the master and duplicate files of written selections, most bibliotherapists need shelf space for filing other materials. The shelf file, for example, would include the multiple copies of a single book used for participant selections; other books, collections, and anthologies that the facilitator regularly consults; and nonprint materials such as phonograph records, cassette tapes, film strips, videocassettes, films, and other odd-sized materials.

Some bibliotherapists keep similar items together and file alphabetically within each category. Others prefer to mix the media and to file in a single alphabet. For print materials, use the author's last name for filing. Then decide on and follow a consistent policy for other media. For example, a film producer is the generally accepted equivalent of an author. But films and other audiovisuals are usually filed by title; in those cases in which a title cannot be found on the container or first frame, supply one of your own. Phonograph records or musical tapes are also difficult to file; decide whether you are likely to remember and locate them by composer, medium, performing artist, or type. You may decide to set up several categories of records. For example, all symphonic music would be filed under the composer in one section, whereas a second grouping of records would include popular music arranged by performer.

It is helpful to hand-letter or type on a gummed label the first three letters of the word according to which the shelved files are being arranged. Attach the label to the spine of each book or to the edges of a container to simplify locating and organizing the materials. Finally, when more than one person is using the resources, keep a record of the policies that are being used.

Indexing bibliotherapeutic materials

Indexes are a facilitator's key to the files. Each item will be indexed in three ways—by author, title, and subject. Some people follow the usual library practice of combining all indexes using a single alphabetical order. However, most bibliotherapists may find it more useful to separate the indexes. Use the system that best suits your work habits but *be consistent.*

For those who do not have background or experience in setting up this kind of file, we will review the format and information included in each index. In general, the information is typed, or neatly printed, on index cards of a uniform size that are kept in a file box (see Figure 6.1). However, those who have access to a personal computer may want to adapt the format to set up disk files. Of course, it is advisable to keep a printout of such files: One should always take precautions against a breakdown in the system that might erase all the data that was so laboriously collected and entered. And, disasters aside, it can be quicker and more convenient to scan a printed sheet for ideas than to look through file by file on the

Lennon, John and Paul McCartney RECORD

"Help!" on The Beatles/1962-1966. Hollywood, CA:

Capitol Industries, Inc. (side 3)

Lyrics in Great Songs of Lennon and McCartney.

1973. New York: Quadrangle/The New York Times Book

Co., pp. 97-99.

To Hell With Dying SHORT STORY

Walker, Alice.

"To Hell With Dying," in

The Best Short Stories by Negro Writers

Langston Hughes, ed. 1967. Boston: Little, Brown

and Co., pp. 490-496.

SELF-AWARENESS

Dobyns, Stephen

"What You Have Come to Expect," The New Yorker,

July 14, 1980. p. 36.

FIGURE 6.1 Examples of index cards: (top) author/title card *for a song from a phonograph record, (center)* title card *for a selection from an anthology, and (bottom)* subject card *for a poem that appeared in a magazine*

screen; then again, someone else may be using the machine, or you may be far from the terminal when you want to look up a reference.

The basic core of information for all three indexes is identical; as only the heading varies, two cards may be typed at once, using carbon paper. This is the form we recommend for the basic information.

1. Indicate the author's name (or that of the editor, compiler, composer, recording artist, producer—depending on the media), last name first, on the fourth line of the card, indented four spaces.
2. On the following line, give the selection title, indented six spaces. If a whole book is being indexed, underline the title. If only one chapter or selection is being noted, put the selection title in quotation marks, followed by the whole book title, underlined.
3. Immediately following the title, give the following bibliographic information: place of publication, publisher, copyright date, and relevant page numbers. Most of these details can be located on either the front or the back of the title page in books. Look on the film can or the slide, filmstrip, tape, videocassette container, or record jacket for the information in other media.
4. On the very top line of the card, in the upper right-hand corner, indicate the format. The usual categories are ARTICLE, FILM, POEM, RECORD, TAPE, SHORT STORY, VIDEOCASSETTE, and so on. Some facilitators who regularly vary the type of material they use prefer to set up a separate *format index* in which all items in one category are filed together alphabetically by author.

Author index cards include the information just indicated and have no special heading other than format information. However, we find it convenient to keep records on this card as well. Accordingly, we separate the author index from the title index and use a larger index card (5 by 7 rather than 3 by 5).

For record-keeping purposes, note the date the material was used, the type of group, and the general nature of the reaction to the material. The record will be more useful if the notation not only indicates whether the group was clinical or developmental but also specifies the exact population (e.g., acute, outpatient, senior citizen, adult women). In addition, try to work out a descriptive set of words to differentiate different reactions. Some possible notations are "thoughtful," "provocative," "produced arguments," "rejected as boring," and "did not elicit personal concerns."

The individual facilitator may find it helpful to evaluate the patterns of response to particular materials. Of course, each group is unique, and the themes and recognitions that emerge in one session will never precisely be duplicated in another. Nonetheless, we have found that some materials invariably stimulate a strong response while others always fall flat. Furthermore, evaluative records compiled from the notes of many different facilitators would be invaluable if someone undertook to research what kind of material worked most effectively in bibliotherapy.

For *title indexes* you can use the usual library format in which the title is retyped on the first line in the upper left-hand corner of the card. However, many facilitators simply underline the title in the second line for their personal files.

Subject indexes include the standard bibliographic information but put the dominant subject or theme in capital letters, centered on the top line of the card. These indexes should be tailored to reflect the needs of the bibliotherapist using them. In particular, use subject headings that are suited to you. For some, that means adopting very precise and detailed categories like those in *Granger's Indexes to Poetry*; others prefer the broader headings used in Leedy (1969) or in Lack (1978). We have found that it is difficult either to settle on or to remember categories that are too finely drawn.

Admittedly, one item may speak to many different themes. Even so, try to impose a limit of no more than two subject cards per selection. Not only will you keep the files down to a manageable size, but you will also find yourself better able to focus on the message of the material.

Some poems, stories, or films are so broad in scope or so universal in application that they cannot easily be categorized. Hence you may end up classifying a great many materials as GENERAL or MULTIFACETED. Other pieces will be classified according to some outstanding feature, such as RHYTHM. This category would include not only literary works such as Poe's "Bells" but other media as well, such as tapes or videocassettes.

Files of complementary materials

In addition to the primary material for a bibliotherapy session, the facilitator may use background music, pictures, photos, art materials, or realia to increase the impact of the text. As your collection of these complementary materials grows, it becomes increasingly important that you file them in a systematic fashion. Some indexing may be desirable as well for large collections. You might also establish separate shelf files for each category of complementary materials, and use the filing and indexing procedure previously indicated for records and tapes.

We shall now look briefly at two other types of complementary materials that bibliotherapists can collect for use.

Picture files. Modern advertising and specialized magazines offer a broad range of photos and illustrations that can be clipped and mounted and then used to increase the impact of bibliotherapeutic material. In addition, art galleries and commercial sources make it possible to acquire reproductions of famous paintings. Pictures of various sizes can be stored in legal-size files or in cardboard file boxes. It is easier to file the names of these pictures word by word than letter by letter, using subject categories. Rather than trying to keep track of many small divisions, use broad categories like FLOWERS, NATURE, PEOPLE, PLACES, TREES, and so on.

Realia files. These files are especially valuable, but they can be awkward. As you will likely spend a good deal of time locating objects that can be used effectively with a given text, you will find it worthwhile to keep such items ready at hand. Use shelves, cupboards, or large boxes to store them, and, although it is not always possible to file alphabetically, be sure to use labels. If the collection becomes extensive or is used by several people, establish and maintain a subject file. A typical set of entries might read ARROWHEADS, BELTS, CAPS-BASEBALL, followed by CAPS-ENGINEERS; it might then continue on through MASKS to XYLOPHONE.

Maintaining files

It is time consuming and sometimes tedious to update all these files and indexes. However, the task is more manageable if you discipline yourself never to allow more than ten items to remain unfiled at any one time. In addition, you should periodically review your collection. Items (particularly complementary materials) that have not been used in some time should be pulled.

The more experience you accumulate, the harder it becomes to accurately remember all of your resources. Accordingly, as time consuming and repetitious as it may seem to maintain three different indexes, it will become increasingly important over time that you have more than one way to retrieve an item.

Selected References for Locating Bibliotherapeutic Materials

To conclude our discussion of bibliotherapeutic materials, we present a list of references that bibliotherapists can use in their search for appropriate and effective materials. The list is not meant to be exhaustive, but it does include some standard library tools. If you are not familiar with any of the items listed, your librarian should be able to guide you as to their location and use.

Note that this list consists primarily of indexes and bibliographic listings for the different genres. We have also included some of the major reference tools for children and adolescent literature, as they contain items that can be used with or adapted to many populations. Note that these citations are not repeated in the final bibliography at the end of the book.

General resources

Books in Print. New York: Bowker, published annually. Three separate listings: *Author, Titles*, and *Subject Guide*. Full publication and ordering information given for each listing. Check for key to abbreviations and addresses for all publishers and distributors.

Chicorel's Indexes. New York: Chicorel Library, published annually. Includes indexes to poetry, poets, anthologies, and short stories.

Reader's Guide to Periodical Literature. New York: Wilson, issued semimonthly and monthly, with bound cumulation issued annually. This author/subject index to selected general interest periodicals also includes references to fiction, poetry, and short stories, and reviews of videodiscs and videotapes.

Poetry

Granger's Indexes to Poetry. Great Neck, N.Y.: Granger's Books. Granger's indexes are based on the anthologies most accessible in small libraries. Citations are not repeated from year to year as the sources tend to go out of print. *Granger's Index to Poetry: 1904 to 1978* covers all volumes that have been indexed in every volume of Granger's and thus provides a listing of the more popular collections of poetry.

Short Stories

Short Story Index. New York: Wilson, 1979. Includes supplements from 1950 to 1978. Alphabetical by author, title, and subject of stories that have appeared in periodicals and collections.

Short Story International. Great Neck, N.Y.: International Cultural Exchange, issued bimonthly. A periodical of unabridged stories. Write to 6 Sheffield Rd., Great Neck, N.Y. 11021

Short Stories in Spanish/Cuentas en español. Miami: Cruzada Spanish Publications, published semiannually. Write to Box 650909, Miami, Fla. 33165.

Fairy tales, folklore, fantasy and science fiction

Clarkson, A., and B. Gilbert. *World Folktales: A Scribner Resource Collection*. New York: Scribner's, 1980. Gives the tale, notes, and comments on principal motifs and parallel stories.

Courlander, H. *A Treasury of Afro-American Folklore: The Oral Literature, Traditions, Recollections, Legends, Tales, Songs, Religious Beliefs, Customs, Sayings, and Humor of People of African Descent in the Americas*. New York: Crown, 1976.

Ireland, N. *Index to Fairy Tales 1949–1972: Including Folklore, Legends, and Myths in Collections*. Westwood, Mass.: F. W. Faxton Co., 1973. Consists of author, title, and subject indexes. (For example, "Cinderella" is one of six tales listed under the subject of Gentleness.)

Schlobin, R. C. *The Literature of Fantasy: A Comprehensive Annotated Bibliography of Modern Fantasy Fiction*. New York: Garland, 1979.

Plays

Plays for Living. New York: Family Service Association of America. (Available on request; write to 44 E. 23rd St., New York, N.Y. 10010.) These one-act thirty-minute plays were developed by a playwright working with experts in the helping professions. They are designed to present current problems, and they are open-ended in order to lead into discussion with the audience. Only five actors are required; sets, costumes, and props are not. The sponsoring organization was begun in 1942 by Katherine Cornell to use live drama to "stimulate new thinking or effect social change" and continues to commission new plays.

Children and adolescent materials

American Library Association. *Subject Index to Poetry for Children and Young People.* Chicago: American Library Association, 1957.

Arbuthnot, M. H., et al. *The Arbuthnot Anthology of Children's Literature.* Glenview, Ill.: Scott, Foresman, 1976.

Arbuthnot, M. H., et al., eds. *Children's Books Too Good to Miss,* 7th ed. New York: University Press Book Service, 1971.

Bernstein, J. *Books to Help Your Children Cope with Separation and Loss,* 2d ed. New York: Bowker, 1983. Annotated author, title, and subject indexes. Interest levels are indicated by subject and ages, and reading levels are indexed by subject and grade.

Carlsen, G. R. *Books and the Teen-age Reader: A Guide for Teachers, Librarians and Parents.* New York: Bantam, 1979. Chapters are devoted to different subject areas with annotated bibliographies.

Children's Books in Print. New York: Bowker, published annually. Author, illustrator, and title indexes for children's fiction and nonfiction (K–12).

Dreyer, S. *The Bookfinder: A Guide to Children's Literature About the Needs and Problems of Youth Aged 12–15.* Circle Pines, Minn.: American Guidance Service, Inc., 1977, 1981. An excellent resource that describes and categorizes children's books by psychological, behavioral, and developmental topics. Includes author and title indexes.

Gillespie, J., and C. Gilbert, eds. *Best Books for Children,* 2d ed. New York: Bowker, 1981. Annotated, by subject.

Index of Poetry for Children and Young People—1970–1975: A Title, Subject, Author, and First-Line Index to Poetry in Collections for Children and Young People. New York: Wilson, 1977.

Kallenbach, J. *Index to Black American Literary Anthologies.* Boston: G. K. Hall, 1979. Listed by author and title.

Polkinghorn, A., and C. Toohey. *Creative Encounters: Activities to Expand Children's Responses to Literature.* Littleton, Colo.: Libraries Unlimited, 1983. Gives synopses of picture books and suggests related stories as well as activities to extend the impact. Some of these activities can be adapted for use as warm-ups or wrap-ups.

Subject Guide to Children's Books in Print. New York: Bowker, published annually.

Tway, E., ed. *Reading Ladders for Human Relations,* 6th ed. Washington, D.C.: American Council on Education, 1981. Author and title index, annotated.

Wilkin, B. T. *Survival Themes in Fiction for Children and Young People.* Metuchen, N.J.: Scarecrow, 1978. A historical survey of book reviews, divided by main subjects: the individual, pairing and grouping, and views of the world.

Periodicals:

Scholastic Magazines, Inc. Englewood Cliffs, N.J., issued periodically throughout the school year. (Write to Magazine Customer Service, 904 Sylvan Ave., Englewood Cliffs, N.J. 07632.) *Voice, Action, Literary Cavalcade,* and *Scope* are magazines containing condensed plays, current television offerings, some poetry, and short stories. All are designed for classroom use, but the topics and themes are also appropriate for older audiences. The length of most of these materials is good for bibliotherapy as well. Multiple copies are available by subscription.

Bulletin for the Center of Children's Books, edited by Zena Sutherland. Chicago: University of Chicago Press, issued monthly. Summarizes and rates new children's books. See also the *School Library Journal,* which contains reviews of current offerings in children's and adolescent books.

Films and other audiovisual materials

Beatty, L. F. *Filmstrips,* vol. 4. Englewood Cliffs, N.J.: Educational Technical Publications (Instructional Media Library), 1981.

Chicorel Index to Poetry in Collections on Discs and Tapes, vol. 4. New York: Chicorel Library, 1972.

Emmens, C. A. *Short Stories on Film.* Littleton, Colo.: Libraries Unlimited, 1978. Indexed by author, followed by the short-story title and film title, a technical description of the film, and an annotation of the film version. Also indexed by short story and film title.

Enser, A. G. *Filmed Books and Plays: A List of Books and Plays from Which Films Have Been Made, 1928–1974,* cumulated ed. New York: Academic Press, 1975. Gives titles of films and authors, titles, and publishers of original materials.

Limbacher, J., ed. *Feature Films on 8mm., 16mm., and Videotape,* 6th ed. New York: Bowker, 1979.

______. *Haven't I Seen You Somewhere Before? Remakes, Sequels, and Series in Motion Pictures and Television, 1896–1978.* Ann Arbor, Mich.: Pierian Press, 1979.

Parlato, S. J. *Films ex Libris: Literature in 16mm. and Video.* Jefferson, N.C.: McFarland and Co., 1979.

Sullivan, K. *Films For, By and About Women.* Metuchen, N.J.: Scarecrow, 1980. Annotated subject index. Lists credits, running time, date, and availability of films.

Periodicals:

Film News. La Salle, Ill.: Open Court Publishing Co., issued quarterly. (Write to Box 619, La Salle, Ill. 61301.) Contains reviews of nontheatrical films and includes feature articles and previews.

Landers Film Reviews. Escondido, Calif.: Landers Association, issued bimonthly. (Write to P.O. Box 27309, Escondido, Calif. 92027.) Provides information on 16mm. films and multimedia materials geared for educational use. This is a monthly title, subject, and source directory, cumulated annually.

Records

Check record stores, which have indexes of currently available records and tapes. Also check music stores for lyrics and sheet music for specific songs.

American Rock and Roll: The Big Hits of the Late 50's and Early 60's, vols. 1 to 6. Ojai, Calif.: Creative Concepts, 1982. Includes sheet music and lyrics. (Write to 967 E. Ojai Ave., Ojai, Calif. 93023.)

Marsh, D., and J. Swenson. *The New Rolling Stone Record Guide*. New York: Rolling Stone Press, 1983. Alphabetical listing of all major rock groups and performers, with information on albums and years issued; brief reviews are included.

Nugent, S., and C. Gillett, eds. *Rock Almanac: Top 20 American and British Singles and Albums of the 50s, 60s and 70s*. New York: Anchor, Doubleday, 1978.

Multisensory Media

Bi-Fokal Productions, Inc. Provides kits for elderly and intergenerational use. (Write to 911 Williamson St., Madison, Wisc. 53703.)

STUDY GUIDE

1. List the main files and indexes that a bibliotherapist would need. Include a brief statement about the value of each.

2. Pick two populations you hope to work with and list the resources mentioned in this chapter that could be used to locate material for each of the groups.

PRACTICUM

1. Identify all the works listed in the "Selected References" section that you are likely to use most often. Make up an additional list of other, related reference materials that you come across and note the special information you can find in each of these materials.

2. Begin your own bibliotherapy files with at least twenty-five items from a variety of genre and media. Decide on the policies you will follow for filing, and record them on index cards to be placed at the front of your file so that you and any other users will be aware of them. Some examples of the policies you might adopt: "Author and title cards to be filed together"; "realia not stored alphabetically"; "classical music filed by composer's name"; "popular music filed separately by performer."

— PART 3 —

THE BIBLIOTHERAPIST

7

Personal Traits of the Bibliotherapist

The facilitator has chosen a Hassidic tale for a bibliotherapy group meeting as part of a university counseling program. The story is very short, and because she feels it will have the most impact if it is told rather than read, she has not prepared a written copy for each participant.

Very briefly, the story is about a certain Lev who dies and goes before the Angel of Judgment. As Lev begins to offer excuses and explanations, the angel interrupts him. "Hold on, Lev," the angel says. "You seem to think I'm going to ask you why you weren't a Moses or an Elijah. But I'm not interested in Moses or Elijah—they've come before me and gone. What I want to know, Lev, is why weren't you Lev—truly Lev, the best Lev you could be?"

When she comes to the end of the story, the bibliotherapist is silent for a minute, letting the material begin its work. She notices one student shifting in his seat and looking as if he has something to say; she nods encouragingly to him. He speaks up. "I don't know about the angel of death," he says, "but my parents sure won't be satisfied unless I'm Moses or Elijah." The first speaker seems reluctant to go on, and the facilitator decides to respect his reticence for the minute. Instead she turns to a person who voiced agreement and invites her to speak. As the girl begins to talk about the pressure she feels from her parents and about her strong sense of inadequacy, the facilitator does not comment much directly but nods or murmurs empathically several times.

As the discussion continues, the facilitator notices that a moody young man has gone from doodling to tapping his pencil on the desk. She tries to draw him into the discussion, but he replies in abrupt monosyllables, and the tapping becomes even more noticeable. The facilitator decides to confront the behavior. Without sounding angry or sarcastic, she says, "Chip, I would really like to know how you feel about this issue. But the way you are responding makes me think you don't want to join in the discussion. That is your right. However, you may not realize the noise from your pencil is making it difficult for those of us who are sharing to concentrate." She lets her attitude indicate that she trusts that Chip will understand and honor a reasonable request and turns to another member with a question.

For the time being, the drumming stops, and the discussion begins to shift from the pressures the students feel from parents and teachers to their explorations of the expectations members have for themselves. This is an issue that the facilitator is personally very aware of. Although she makes a few remarks, she is careful not to dominate the discussion or to drive home forcefully various principles she feels the young people could benefit from—she respects the need and the right they have to learn such irretrievably personal lessons for themselves.

The facilitator had intended to spend the last part of the session in having each participant draw a picture or write a poem about his or her "real" self. However, the students have been very involved in the discussion, and the time is almost up. Even Chip has volunteered a few remarks. Instead of trying to force her plan, the facilitator adapts to the needs and interests of the group and allows the dialogue to continue to the end of the period.

A BIBLIOTHERAPIST SHOULD DEMONSTRATE the necessary therapeutic attitudes of empathy, respect, and genuineness. These attitudes grow out of the personal characteristics of maturity, integrity, adaptability, and responsibility. It is important to clarify how we understand these qualities and the roles they play.

Empathy

Empathy is defined as the capacity to understand intellectually or imaginatively another's feelings or thoughts without actually experiencing them oneself. For the bibliotherapist, this quality involves both the ability to *perceive* accurately what the participant feels and means and the capacity to *communicate* back to the participant an understanding and an acceptance of the other's private inner feelings and thoughts. Although not all theories of therapeutic communication stress empathy, we agree, for example, with that of Carkhuff (1969), who sees empathy as the variable "from which all other dimensions flow in the helping process."

Accurate perceptions

Empathy is based on evidence, not on presumptions. The facilitator is careful to listen for what is actually communicated rather than assuming that a certain response will be given or reading much more into the comments than is actually there. Particularly in cases in which a facilitator has been working with a participant for a time and has a good sense of his or her interests and needs, it is important not to anticipate a reaction before the individual actually makes it.

On the other hand, Reik (1949) speaks of the empathic "third ear," which permits the facilitator to use both intuition and sensitivity to subtle cues to help the participants deal with submerged issues that they may not as yet recognize. Similarly, Bandler and Grinder (1975) speak of the importance of listening for the "deep structure" of what is expressed, rather than settling for "surface structure" messages.

The process of getting the participants to specify precisely what they understand and feel can demand a great deal of empathic skill and time. Some clinical or developmental participants will have little previous experience in being precise to draw on; others will actively resist exploring their own realities in any meaningful way. It is important for the bibliotherapist to facilitate the habit of reflection and to persuade participants to overcome their resistance to the degree that is appropriate. However, it is equally vital that confrontation not be forced on a fragile personality. In effect, a good bibliotherapist is able to distinguish between true empathy and the basically narcissistic need to dazzle or to present an interpretation with which the individual is not ready to cope.

The facilitator bases empathic understanding on both verbal and nonverbal messages. It is important to check frequently with participants about the meaning of their verbal responses. As we have indicated, the facilitator should work at reflecting back as accurately as possible what the participant said, rather than attempting to interpret hidden meanings.

But it is also important to check on nonverbal messages. Blushes, frowns, and looks of shock and dismay as well as expressions of relief or pleasure all seem quite clear. Posture, tone of voice, and eye contact may suggest a response when nothing is said. For example, stiff movements, slouching, turning away from another, or an aggressive stance can all be read by a sensitive observer to indicate tension or hostility. Tapping one's fingers or foot, doodling, fussing with one's hair, or biting one's nails are signs of boredom or anxiety. By the same token, the expression in one's eyes can convey warmth and regard, amusement, indifference, coldness, or dislike.

As significant as such nonverbals are, however, it is essential that the facilitator "read" them in terms of the individual involved. Schizophrenics frequently have uncommunicative faces, for example, and many other persons have learned to discipline how they look. Although posture is usually telling, some people force themselves to look relaxed even when they are feeling extreme tension. So, too, there are individuals whose voices are softest when they are most angry or whose habitual tone is abrasive even when they are being friendly or helpful. Bibliotherapists learn to check the accuracy of their interpretations with the participants themselves with remarks like "You look as if what was just said upset you; would you like to comment?" or "You seem to find today's material boring. Shall we talk about what makes it so unappealing to you?"

Clearly, it is not easy to understand accurately another's feelings and responses. Empathy seems to be something of a natural gift that can be developed and used more therapeutically through training and practice (Hoffman 1965). Thus, even though good supervision probably cannot turn a rigid, intolerant person into an empathic facilitator, it can help someone who is naturally other-directed learn what to look for. As supervisors go over written or verbal replays of the session, watch videotapes, observe through a one-way mirror, or sit in on a session, they look for cues from the participants that the trainee missed or misread, or they suggest alternative ways of handling a response or situation.

Communicating empathy

One of the qualities the supervisor looks for most carefully is the accuracy and effectiveness of the facilitator's empathic responses. It is just as important that the bibliotherapist know how to communicate understanding and acceptance as it is to accurately interpret what the participant means.

Beginning bibliotherapists in particular may need help from an observer and from self-critiquing through videotapes to become aware of the nonverbal messages *they themselves are sending*. Participants may consciously or unconsciously read the facilitator's tone of voice or body language as an indication of shock, dislike, indifference, rejection, or negative judgment. Since participants usually do not comment or check the accuracy of their perceptions of these nonverbal messages, the bibliotherapist must be very conscious of his or her tone, posture, gestures, eye movements, and expression and of how these might be interpreted—or misinterpreted.

In general, bibliotherapists find that a quiet, almost matter-of-fact attitude is the most convincing. Tone of voice and the expression in one's eyes are important ways to indicate warmth and interest. Effusive behavior can frighten or threaten some people; others are made uneasy by overly familiar gestures such as hugging or touching. More often than not, a quiet assumption that members will respect proper behavioral boundaries is successful, whereas an ultimatum or show of annoyance might cause resistance.

A truly empathic facilitator communicates that his or her understanding is both accurate and nonjudgmental. The implicit message is "I understand that you are feeling this way (for instance, angry, sad, or helpless). I am acknowledging the reality of your emotion and the need you have to deal with it independent of whether or not I share your reaction or feel that the response is appropriate or proportionate." The empathic facilitator may or may not feel sympathetic, but pity is not a therapeutic response. As we understand it, pity stems from a conviction of superiority; the other person is seen as trapped by circumstances or emotions that he or she is not capable of overcoming. Basically, we feel that the facilitator who pities or reproaches the participant instead of conveying understanding and acceptance also will not demonstrate respect—the second fundamental quality of a good bibliotherapist.

Respect

In many ways, respect is another facet of empathy. Yet there is a real distinction between the two. It is possible to be empathic (that is, to accurately perceive and communicate back another's feelings) without having respect for the individual (that is, without valuing both the feelings and the inherent worth and uniqueness of the other individual).

But the obverse is equally true. Sometimes it is not possible to understand an individual well enough to perceive accurately what that person feels. Even so, the facilitator can communicate his or her profound belief that all people have inherent worth and are uniquely capable of making decisions and of working through their own growth. More than that, the facilitator can make it clear that he or she does not regard the participants as being somehow inherently inferior—that is, as the "they" out there who have problems totally unrelated to any the facilitator might experience. Rather, a good facilitator recognizes that the human condition is a common denominator we all share.

Respect versus the savior complex

Genuine respect means that the bibliotherapist does not confuse helping someone help themselves with "saving" the other (more often than not, the rationale is to "save him from himself"). On the contrary, a good facilitator recognizes that a savior attitude is fundamentally demeaning, as it postulates that the person being saved is of diminished worth and not capable of real growth. Second, the savior tends to create a dependency in the other that can both perpetuate unhealthy coping patterns and block the self-affirmation that comes from working out a problem for oneself. Finally, as valuable and as stimulating as good facilitation can be, no emotional problem or issue can be resolved unless the individual participant personally works at and integrates a solution that is uniquely appropriate to him or her.

Like others in the mental-health field, the bibliotherapist must regularly assess his or her individual motives with respect to "saving" participants. Those who find themselves concentrating on materials that will bring out problem areas and tending to favor dialogues that probe difficulties rather than examine and affirm strengths should consider carefully whether they truly respect the participants or whether, instead, they are more concerned with satisfying their own egos by "solving" others' problems.

In short, respect has a double function in relation to the bibliotherapist. Not only is it important to show respect for the participants, it is also part of the bibliotherapist's task to facilitate the participant's sense of mutuality and respect for others.

Ultimately, then, for both facilitator and participant, showing respect is a therapeutic act. Erikson cautions us that someone who never attends to others can "suffer the mental deformation of self-absorption, in which he becomes his own infant and pet" (1964, 130). On the other hand, Erikson points out, mutuality "strengthens the doer even as it strengthens the other."

Communicating respect

Exercising and communicating respect are skills that all bibliotherapists must work at as they choose materials; respond to participants' remarks, insights, or opinions; and utilize what emerges in the dialogue. In the course of a session, the facilitator indicates his or her respect for the individual group members through both verbal and nonverbal clues that make it clear that each person's contribution is valued. A bibliotherapist always listens attentively to everyone—both to those who speak readily and to those who need to be drawn out. The facilitator's tone of voice, bearing, and gestures should help communicate that all verbal and written responses are considered to be worthy of serious consideration. Even when the facilitator finds it necessary to tell participants that they are not speaking in a way that can be understood, he or she must do so in a respectful way.

We will go into more detail about specific strategies for respectfully facilitating a bibliotherapy session in subsequent chapters. But we can indicate here a few examples of responses that are disrespectful. First, the bibliotherapist who is too directive often bypasses or fails to hear responses that do not fit a preconceived agenda. Furthermore, it is essential that the facilitator respect and trust the participants' capacity to see something unique and meaningful in the material. Moreover, although the facilitator may find it necessary to firmly cut off someone who is overvocal, perseverating, or clearly manipulating, it is never appropriate to do so scornfully or in a way that belittles the individual. On the other hand, it is equally wrong to force disclosures. The bibliotherapist must always respect the individual's right not to pursue an issue.

Second, we have mentioned the healing potential of humor—but the bibliotherapist must scrupulously avoid anything that would suggest to a participant that he or she is being laughed at or made fun of. Above all, the facilitator must be very aware of the vulnerability and risk involved in honestly revealing and dialoguing about feeling-responses. Any misuse of the revealed material would be not only disrespectful but a serious violation of the bibliotherapist's responsibilities as well.

Genuineness

Empathy and respect, the first two qualities fundamental to a bibliotherapist discussed thus far, concern the way the bibliotherapist relates to the participants. But the third quality, genuineness, bears on the way the bibliotherapist sees self. Effective facilitators are comfortable with themselves; they are sincere and capable of being spontaneous and open. They recognize that they must do what they are asking the participants to do: to be aware of inner experiences, to be honest about them, and to claim them as their own. At the same time, they are free enough not to impose their personal feelings on others.

In a sense, then, genuineness creates the balance necessary for healthy empathy and respect. A genuine person can distinguish between the participant's actual responses and the facilitator's temptation to read meaning into what is said. At the same time, genuineness allows the facilitator to see how the expressed feelings might reflect psychic problems, yet leaves him or her to empathize at the same time. There is no need to put others down or to make them unhealthily dependent. Hence the facilitator must not fall into using materials or making interventions that are well meant but inappropriate.

Self-awareness

In effect, bibliotherapists who are genuine are also self-aware. They know themselves well enough to be able to put their own needs aside so that they can listen accurately to the participants. A facilitator can never be fully effective without this quality. It is like someone listening to Mahler's "Fourth Symphony" on a radio with reception trouble. As the tuning deteriorates, Mahler is blurred and distorted by interference from the neighboring rock-and-roll station. In the same way, the internal rhythms of a bibliotherapist who is unaware of or preoccupied by self will distort or block out the verbal and nonverbal responses of the participants.

Real harm can be done when the facilitator fails to explore precisely whose needs and interests are being served by the choice of material and direction of the dialogue. Helen DeRosis makes this point well in her guidelines to psychotherapists:

> You may believe that your patient wants to return to his mother's womb, but how would it help him to discuss his dependency in those terms? Is it, further, of

any help to him to discuss his dependency at all? Or might this only add to an already abiding sense of inadequacy as a human being? If you do insist, however, upon discussing this point with him, and he finally agrees with you, what does he do then? Does he try to climb back in, or does he remain forever frustrated and furious that this is impossible? . . .

What, then, is to be the content of a therapeutic session, whether individual or group? Undoubtedly pathology will be talked about, but it would seem that equal or greater emphasis might be placed upon talking about and/or experiencing the healthy features of the patient's character structure, environment, and development. To discover, identify, and describe these features may take greater skill than to deal with pathology. (1978, 6)

There is a critical difference between leading a discussion without experiencing personal reactions and doing so without allowing personal reactions to intrude. In other words, a facilitator who is appropriately genuine has emotions or needs but is able to recognize them and, beyond that, is able and willing to take into account how such reactions may affect interactions with the participants.

For example, a trainee was counseled after a session during which she encouraged rather than cut off a rather raucous discussion in which a group of disturbed adolescent boys tried to turn the focus to sexual innuendos in Edwin Morgan's very aggressive poem "Hyena." The choice of material and the facilitation of the meeting suggest that this trainee had not yet come to terms with the limitations of her own role—she did not have the experience or training to qualify her to deal therapeutically with the very complex sexual issues troubling a number of the group members. If nothing else, given the nature of the group, both the choice of material and direction of the dialogue could have erupted into a physically threatening situation. In any case, such problems are better addressed over a period of time in a one-on-one situation rather than in passing within a group.

It is not possible to distinguish the responses that come from within from those based on accurate observation of the participants until the facilitator recognizes his or her own feelings of frustration, boredom, fear of approaching a certain subject, or even personal dislike for a particular member of a group. Yet a simple acknowledgment of the feeling is sometimes enough to stop it from interfering with empathy and respect. For example, one might say, "I know I find this person's constant sulkiness very irritating; but let me look beyond my reaction so that I can attend to the exact messages he is sending about today's material."

On occasion, it is necessary to express a negative reaction to a group member's behavior. But such a message should be both genuine and respectful. For example, the facilitator could say to a member who continually refuses to share any response to the literature, "I find myself being uneasy when you don't say anything because I feel helpless to help you," or "I have been trying to find things that interest you. Could you help me by mentioning some topics you might like?" Both of these remarks avoid placing blame on the participant at the same time that they show concern for him. In other words, the point of the intervention is not to vent the facilitator's irritation—however justified it may be—but to communicate to the participant that his or her needs are primary.

In some cases the facilitator might need supervisory or therapeutic help to deal with an issue. For example, one bibliotherapist found that she became very uneasy and tried to bypass responses that looked as though they might lead to discussion of death or suicide. After talking with her supervisor, she decided that it was best to use material in which these themes were very unlikely to arise until she could get professional help in working out some of the unresolved issues that made it so difficult for her to dissociate her own reactions from any discussion of these subjects.

Expressing genuineness

As we have noted, genuineness concerns the bibliotherapist's attitude toward self—but there are several areas in which the need to be genuine must be weighed against other demands. For instance, facilitators can legitimately look for items whose style, form, or presentation appeal to their personal taste. But some people who come to bibliotherapy from backgrounds in literature find it hard to use any works that they find of dubious aesthetic value. It is not always practical or advantageous to fully indulge personal tastes in this way. It may be necessary to work at allowing other dimensions to outweigh poetic value.

For example, we consider John Donne to be immeasurably superior to Edwin Markham as a poet. Yet many, many more participants will be able to respond meaningfully to Markham's "Outwitted," a four-line poem about the circle drawn by love, than to Donne's magnificent but abstruse "Valediction Concerning Mourning," which also plays on the theme of love's encompassing circle. Sometimes the bibliotherapist will choose to spend many extra hours finding a "good" poem that treats the critical theme in a way that most participants will respond to. But in time, those with high aesthetic standards can become "genuine" while using a poem like "Outwitted" because they have learned to differentiate between good literature and literature that is good for bibliotherapy.

The bibliotherapist must also work out a proper balance between sharing his or her genuine feeling-response and not intruding into the therapeutic dialogue. There is no absolute rule for deciding on the best strategy: The facilitator must call on empathy and experience to determine the approach that is most helpful in a given situation. At times, the participant benefits from being aware of the facilitator as someone who shares a feeling-response to the material or dialogue. At other times, the facilitator's own reaction to the discussion may be intrusive or even intimidating to the members.

During training, the bibliotherapist's supervisor will regularly raise questions that involve genuineness. Again, both the trainee and the supervisor will usually find it easier to critique while watching a video or listening to a taped replay than they possibly could while the session was actually going on.

Personal Characteristics

As previously noted, the fundamental therapeutic attitudes we have just described grow out of the bibliotherapist's personal maturity, integrity, sense of responsibility, and adaptability. As we look at the way each of these qualities affects the bibliotherapist's capability, keep in mind that we are not speaking of characteristics that a potential trainee should anticipate acquiring. Rather, these are qualities that must be present from the outset. The training is meant only to increase the effectiveness with which they are demonstrated.

Although it may seem presumptuous to insist on the required profile, in fact we are only asking that those who facilitate bibliotherapy be actively engaged in the same process of growth and self-affirmation in which they are guiding the participants and that they be capable of relating effectively to others.

Maturity

In the sense that we understand it, maturity is a function not of age but of an attitude toward self in relation to others. In effect, maturity is a prerequisite for empathy and respect and is a necessary complement to genuineness. The mature person is not only self-aware; he or she is self-accepting and, correspondingly, tolerant of others as well. Able to stand outside of a situation and to be amused at what is absurd in oneself, such an individual accepts his or her personal fallibility and neither fears nor avoids working toward personal growth.

Keeping oneself in perspective frees the mature person from crippling self-absorption and thus makes it possible for the individual to demonstrate the unselfishness, patience, perseverance, and sense of one's own limits necessary to practice effective bibliotherapy. Hence a mature person does not agonize unnecessarily over a session that went poorly. There are always those days when things do not go well. The individuals in the group will work on their needs at their own rates, not necessarily in accord with the facilitator's timetable.

Indeed, particularly with clinical groups, the facilitator may have to exercise a great deal of perspective not to be discouraged as week after week schizophrenics simply shriek or engage in a steady stream of "word-salad" remarks, or as depressed patients fail to speak or respond only to let the facilitator know that it is almost time for dinner. But even when a group is in fairly good control and members are actively participating, the facilitator must still be mature enough to tolerate mundane and repetitious discussions, semi-articulate explanations, resistance, and/or acting-out behaviors. Above all, the bibliotherapist must be able to go without the gratification of clear and immediate results. More often than not, the process of growth is slow and almost imperceptible.

In any case, although mature bibliotherapists appropriately find some gratification in demonstrating competency and in seeing indications that they have contributed to another's well-being, they never make personal satisfaction their primary goal. Indeed, maturity informs the bibliotherapist's fundamental conviction that each individual is responsible only for self and that as important as it is to help, one is ultimately unable to save another. The literature and the guided dialogue are only tools that each individual in the group may or may not choose to use for personal growth and/or healing. In short, the effective and competent bibliotherapist has the maturity to accept that "the things we love we have to learn to leave alone."

Integrity

Integrity goes hand in hand with maturity. Bibliotherapists should consciously work from a personally integrated moral framework. The inherent respect they have for themselves as well as for others means that they will have the integrity to avoid compromising their own principles or self-esteem as well as to reject anything that would lead to exploiting another. In other words, bibliotherapists must scrupulously avoid playing upon emotions, forcing anyone to disclose more than he or she is comfortable with revealing, taking advantage of information that has emerged, or pressuring participants into needlessly extended therapy.

Responsibility

The maturity and integrity of successful bibliotherapists ensures that they will understand and meet the responsibilities of their role. We will look at the procedural obligations in the next chapter, but here we can briefly note the equally serious implications that a sense of responsibility has for the bibliotherapist's attitudes.

In the first place, the facilitator must be responsible in the root sense of the word—"to act in return," or "to react positively or cooperatively." He or she is responsible not only for eliciting feeling-responses but, more particularly, for helping the participants understand those emotions and achieve some kind of closure. We have stressed how critical it is that the bibliotherapist should not force a confrontation the individual is not ready for. However, it is equally important that participants are helped to genuinely probe their feeling-responses and to continue the process of growth even when it is uncomfortable or painful. In the context of strategies for facilitating (Chapter 9), we will look more closely at how the bibliotherapist exercises the responsibility for respectful and sensitive challenging of the participants.

Yet bibliotherapists have obligations to themselves and to their profession concurrent with those they owe the group members. In particular, those intending to enter this field will see the need to accept guidance and supervision as they learn the theory and practice the skills necessary for bibliotherapy. Someone who refuses to listen to advice and to honestly evaluate his or her understanding and performance lacks the respect and genuineness necessary to lead others in a similar growth process.

Of course, the need to be professional and to work constantly at maintaining and improving skills does not stop at the end of training but continues as long as a person practices bibliotherapy.

Adaptability

Adaptability is somewhat different from the other qualities we have identified as being necessary for a bibliotherapist. To begin with, this quality is much more neutral in a moral sense. In addition, adaptability is both less dependent on and less reflective of maturity than are integrity or a sense of responsibility.

Even so, this quality is essential in at least three major ways. First, a bibliotherapist must be comfortable with the fact that nothing is assured before a group or individual session begins. Although it is important to think out possible interventions if the material does not spontaneously spark a response, effective bibliotherapy depends on the fact that the potential always exists for a unique interaction between the literature and the participant. The bibliotherapist who draws up and tries to carry out a preconceived plan will be so focused on measuring how the actual responses compare to the intended direction that he or she will not be able to listen accurately and effectively to the group members' reactions.

Second, the facilitator must be responsive to the "present moment" of the individual or individuals in the group. Since catharsis, self-application, and integration cannot be programmed, the bibliotherapist must be prepared to maximize skillfully the effect of such responses when they are triggered by something in the material or dialogue. At times, it is necessary to abruptly shift the direction of the discussion to take full advantage of one member's sudden recognition. At other times, the facilitator will have to decide quickly on a new strategy to deal with an unexpected resistance. Obviously, even the most experienced bibliotherapists will miss some of these critical moments;

but someone who anticipates a certain response or is not flexible enough to switch strategies will regularly fail to take advantage of the present moment.

Third, the skilled bibliotherapist is not so invested in the meaning that he or she personally finds in the material that the participants are blocked from interpreting it for themselves. Thus the facilitator must be adaptable enough to let stand a misreading of the text if it is clear that the message the participant discovered could lead to self-understanding. As we have indicated, those with a strong background in analyzing and explicating literature may have trouble adapting to the much looser approach necessary for bibliotherapy. For example, we have found that poets and writers who are bibliotherapists usually find it impossible to dissociate themselves sufficiently from their own work to effectively facilitate its use.

STUDY GUIDE

1. Choose one of the fundamental therapeutic attitudes (empathy, respect, genuineness) and analyze the degree to which this attitude is based on the personal qualities of maturity, integrity, responsibility, and adaptability.

2. Discuss the reasons for which a "savior" attitude is not therapeutic.

3. Look up and report on one or more of the following readings in terms of how it bears on effective facilitating in bibliotherapy. In a classroom, ask students to present their reports in a panel format. (a) Report on Jourard (1964, 59–65; 121–132), whose work is especially relevant to nurses or others in helping professions; (b) report on the summary chapter of Hammond et al. (1978, 333–349), which concerns the use of Carl Roger's person-centered therapy; (c) for discussions of nonverbal behaviors in a therapeutic setting, read Berger (1975), D'Augelli et al. (1980, 13–18), Gendlin (1971), Knapp (1980), or Remacker and Storch (1982); (d) report on the concept of the "third ear" (Reik 1949); (e) use Applebaum (1966) as the basis for a report on evocativeness and rapport; (f) report on Carkhuff's guidelines for communicating empathy, respect, and genuineness (1969, 201–213).

PRACTICUM

As the following series of exercises is longer than most, extra time may have to be scheduled to ensure that each trainee experiences each of the three traits (empathy, respect, and genuineness). It is also important that future bibliotherapists get some experience with the basic therapeutic attitudes before working with participants. If at all possible, videotape the first set of exercises to be used with the second set.

1. Divide the class into pairs for role-playing. In each case, arrange to reverse roles for the role-playing. Allow 20 minutes for role-playing, 15 minutes in which both partners discuss together how the attitude was or could be demonstrated, and 15 minutes in which both make a list of the ways in which the understandings gained from the experience could be applied to bibliotherapy. In the first team, one person will try to demonstrate *accurate empathy* in a situation in which the other person has been surprised while he or she is weeping. In the second team, one person will assume the role of showing *respect* to the other, who will vehemently express anger in rough language. In the third team, one person will try to be *genuine* in response to a situation in which the other will unexpectedly express resentment over a past situation that the two had shared. Finally, a committee from the class will prepare a summary of the techniques and qualities compiled from the lists made up by the different teams.

2. Devote several sessions to studying the videotapes made in the first exercise. First, view and analyze different examples of how empathy was shown; at another time, concentrate on respect and then on genuineness.

FURTHER READINGS

Rogers (1957 and 1966) succinctly states his basic approach, known as person-centered therapy. Rogers and Dymond (1978) have edited articles on bringing about personality changes through psychotherapy. Weigart (1960 and 1961) sensitively analyzes loneliness, trust, and sympathy in the art of psychotherapy. Hammond et al. (1978) offer an excellent textbook on therapeutic communication that includes very useful exercises. Full chapters are devoted to developing empathy, respect, and genuineness. Watzlawick (1978) is another good presentation of the elements of therapeutic communication.

Horney (1945, 1950) includes a discussion of the need for care in forcing confrontations, whereas Goleman (1979) provides a short, popularized presentation of Lazarus's theory that there can be psychic value in what he terms "positive denial." For a fuller discussion, see Lazarus (1966, 1974). Finally, Havens's (1974) existential practice of "being and staying" is somewhat similar to Rogers's approach but can usefully be applied to bibliotherapy.

8

The Bibliotherapist's Responsibilities

When the library board of a medium-sized city announced that it wanted to see more community involvement, a branch librarian got permission to include bibliotherapy services as part of her job description. She planned to continue the two developmental groups she had been running for over a year: a poetry club made up primarily of housewives and retirees and a mothers' group that met at the same time as a preschoolers' story hour.

Now the librarian could work on doing something with the residents of a nearby halfway house for discharged mental patients. The librarian recognized that she did not have a mandate to work with these people one-on-one, but she believed that a bibliotherapy group would be an appropriate way to involve the residents in the library. She contacted the social worker associated with the halfway house and began to work out details of recruitment and screening. She also discussed how long each session should be and the most advantageous time of day and location. They decided to begin by using a small conference room in the library.

The social worker agreed to help "remind" the participants to show up for the first several sessions, scheduled for early in weekday afternoons. The librarian was careful to be visible near the front of the library on these days so that she could greet the group members and show them to the room. She also asked the social worker to critique tapes of several sessions and to suggest further readings that would help her understand and deal with the needs of this population.

As the various groups began to meet regularly, the librarian found that the procedures for each group varied. For example, the timing of the young mothers' group was closely tied to the story hour; since the conference room was not available then, the group had to meet in a corner of the main reading room. Although there were some distractions, the group was small and the members were very motivated to use literature as another source of insight into the problems of parenting young children. The librarian was about the same age and shared many interests with these women—she herself had a three-year-old son. Everyone was comfortable on a first-name basis. The poetry group, too, had grown up on its own, and the members were on terms of easy familitarity.

However, the atmosphere in the newly established group was much more formal. The librarian noticed that many of the participants had introduced themselves as Mr. or Mrs., rather than by a first name; she felt it was important to respect this convention. The small-room setting did cut down outside distractions, but the librarian found that she had to spend much more time in raising awareness of the rights and needs of other members and in working out procedural issues such as policies for coming in late or leaving early.

By the end of six months, however, all of the groups were operating quite smoothly, and the librarian and her superiors were talking enthusiastically about adding a senior citizens' group.

IN THIS CHAPTER WE EXAMINE the responsibility the bibliotherapist has for working out procedures and logistics and the issues each such decision involves.

General Procedural Decisions

Most potential bibliotherapists begin with some sense of whether they would be interested in a one-on-one dialogue or a group structure as well as with some idea of the type of participant they are likely to work with, at least initially. Even then, however, both of these choices reflect a decision among valid alternatives.

The format

The decision as to whether the bibliotherapeutic dialogue will take place between the facilitator and the participant on a one-on-one basis or in a group setting depends on several factors including training, personal preference, and practical considerations.

Many licensed psychotherapists have preferred to use the familiar therapist-to-client approach in bibliotherapy (see Leedy 1969, 1973; Lerner 1978; Schloss 1976). Other bibliotherapists find the group approach effective. Either mode is acceptable, but the important thing is that the individual bibliotherapist be trained in and comfortable with the mode he or she is using. In developmental as well as clinical bibliotherapy, it is often simply more economical and more efficient to use a group structure. Since this format is by far more common in any case, we will assume in much of the following discussion that the procedural and logistical issues are being dealt with in the context of a group.

The contract

The nature of the agreement between the bibliotherapist and the participant depends upon the mode of interactive bibliotherapy being used. Every clinical bibliotherapist makes an explicit commitment to use the tool of literature for therapeutic healing. The exact nature of the contract, however, varies according to circumstances. For example, psychotherapists who use clinical bibliotherapy in a one-on-one format with a client will work out a verbal or written contract that indicates general or specific goals, the frequency and number of sessions, and the financial arrangements. Such a contract would be modified for private clients in a group setting.

Somewhat different terms apply to clinical bibliotherapy in institutional settings such as mental hospitals, community health centers, or correctional institutions (Hinseth 1975). Since bibliotherapy is carried on as one part of the treatment program of the institution, only rarely would there be a written contract for this particular mode. However, the participants do have a right to be informed of the general goals and expectations as well as the frequency and initial duration of the sessions. A discussion of these issues should be held within the group. In ongoing sessions in which some participants regularly move to outpatient status and others join the group as they enter the unit, the facilitator should still ensure that each new member is aware of the nature of this particular therapy.

For the most part, there is no need for a formal contract between the participant and facilitator in a developmental group. However, all parties involved should work out an agreement about the general goals and the initial policy for timing and setting. Once again, note that a developmental bibliotherapist has an implicit contract only to further normal growth and understanding. Participants can expect to improve self-esteem and to work out such common issues as the meaning of anger or the ambivalence many people feel about their close relatives (i.e., siblings, parents, or children).

As even normal growth can be painful, the developmental bibliotherapist should expect to have to work at times to overcome resistance. However, it is virtually never appropriate for a bibliotherapist to take on such devastating problems as suicide, chronic depression, self-hate, or serious delusions within the developmental bibliotherapy group setting. Not only do most developmental bibliotherapists lack the training to deal as the primary therapist with such issues, but it is seldom in the best interests of the individual or the group as a whole to focus on such serious problems in this setting. Rather, the individual should be referred for qualified help.

Selection and Screening: Clinical Bibliotherapy

As the procedures for recruiting and screening clinical participants are different from those used with developmental groups, each mode will be discussed separately.

Selection

Psychotherapists working with individual clients may either regularly use interactive bibliotherapy or decide that this approach is particularly appropriate for a given person. In both instances, the therapist is responsible for seeing that the client is willing to try the mode and likely to benefit from it.

In institutional settings, bibliotherapy is likely to be one of a number of scheduled therapeutic activities. Depending on current standards of practice, the facilitator may be present at treatment-planning meetings in which decisions are made as to which individuals are available and likely to benefit from a given therapy. Interactive bibliotherapy groups may be organized to meet in particular wards such as those designated for admissions, chronic patients, or forensic (criminally insane) populations. Alternatively, bibliotherapy may be scheduled as one of several off-the-ward options that patients may choose. In the latter case, meetings might take place in the hospital library or in some other designated location.

Groups established through mixed wards or offered as an open choice can include participants suffering from a wide range of mental illnesses and displaying a variety of behaviors. Although this almost random grouping is not optimal, it may be necessary for organizational reasons. If the range of variation is too great, the facilitator may wish to schedule more workable groupings, such as separating schizophrenics with strong delusional behavior from persons suffering from severe depression.

Nonetheless, participants are likely to show different degrees of pathology and patterns of behavior in all clinical groups. A certain amount of heterogeneity is not only inevitable; often it is productive as well. Even so, it is generally unwise to have one obvious minority member, such as one young person in a group of elderly patients, one woman in an otherwise all male group, or one handicapped person in a group of physically able persons.

Size

Seven to nine members seems to be a good size for groups whose members are consistently present. On the one hand, each member will be able to test ideas against a productive variety of backgrounds and orientations. On the other hand, the number is small enough to ensure that everyone will have a chance to participate and that specific issues can be examined in sufficient depth in the course of a session.

Because of the variety of circumstances that affect attendance or participation, many clinical groups have a somewhat larger total membership than the optimum. For example, groups that include one or two very withdrawn members, or one or two who are often late or absent, might enroll a total of ten or twelve to ensure that there will be six or eight active participants in any given session. Open wards and prison groups are especially likely to have fluctuating attendance owing to medical or legal appointments, visits, or other unexpected circumstances. Even with a total of twelve to fifteen members, such groups on some days will have only four or five participants.

In some long- and short-term drug or alcohol programs, the size of the group can be much larger than is usually considered workable. For example, the fifteen to twenty-five members typically enrolled in residential rehabilitative programs often have a very cohesive attitude about their group. Indeed, we have found it possible to work very effectively with groups of this size. Here, too, the bibliotherapy sessions build on the dialoguing skills and the emphasis on self-evaluation that characterize all aspects of these highly structured programs.

Screening

Even though the initiative for enrolling an individual in a clinical bibliotherapy group usually comes from the ward administrator, psychologist, or treatment team rather than from the patient, the bibliotherapist should schedule a screening interview with each potential participant. The personal interview allows the facilitator to inform the patients about what is likely to happen in the bibliotherapy group and to let the patient come to see the facilitator as a potential helper and as a person to be trusted.

Most persons will respond to an empathic facilitator's invitation to join the clinical bibliotherapy group with at least begrudging acceptance. Those who have trouble reading or who suffer from handicaps should be assured that their difficulties will be accommodated. The bibliotherapist should emphasize that even though reading is involved, the sessions are not like a class in which skills or knowledge are tested. Virtually anyone interested and willing to work on a feeling-response can participate successfully.

In fact, the only real impediment to membership in a clinical group is the wrong attitude. Those who show downright anger or severe withdrawal when entry is suggested may not be suited to this mode. The decision to exclude, however, should be made in consultation with other members of the treatment team, as more than one attempt may be required to reach a deeply hostile or aggressive individual.

We have found that the screening interviews are more successful if they are done in a low-key rather than formal manner. A couple of weeks before the actual group is scheduled to meet, the bibliotherapist visits the ward(s) on which the patients live. The initial contact is one-on-one, even though actual bibliotherapy will be in a group setting. The facilitator can introduce him- or herself to a potential member and ask if they might talk together briefly. In the course of this discussion, the facilitator first explains that a bibliotherapy group is being planned and that the individual has been suggested as a member, and then describes what is involved in participation.

We have found it helpful to bring along a variety of magazines or paperback books to help initiate these conversations. The material gives a concrete indication of the basic tool that will be used in bibliotherapy. In addition, the potential member's response to the items will usually indicate something about his or her interests.

In short, the screening interview has the second important function of allowing the bibliotherapist to learn personal data and general personality information that will provide an accurate basis for (1) making the initial bibliotherapy report; (2) anticipating which of the bibliotherapeutic goals seem to be most applicable to this individual; (3) choosing relevant material once the group actually begins; and (4) establishing the groundwork for future evaluation of progress.

Because the initial interview can be taxing for all and, for that matter, may not be sufficient to cover all the necessary points, it is a good practice to follow up with two or three additional informal visits to the location at which the bibliotherapy program is scheduled to begin. Once there, the bibliotherapist greets all who are present on the ward but actually visits with those scheduled to participate in the bibliotherapy group. Again, it is prudent to bring along paperbacks or magazines to provide some focus for conversation.

The procedures we have just outlined describe how to start up a new clinical bibliotherapy group. Once a group is functioning, however, other potential members may move onto the ward or be referred in some other way. The bibliotherapist, in that instance, is responsible for contacting and interviewing these persons before they formally join the group.

Recruitment and Screening: Developmental Bibliotherapy

Recruitment

The context in which a developmental bibliotherapy group is organized usually determines the way in which members are recruited. Groups organized as part of a church, community, or library program will use the sponsoring organization to help publicize and attract members. A general invitation to an introductory meeting might be posted on a bulletin board or included in church bulletins or community newsletters. In some cases, the pastor, rabbi, librarian, or community worker will know individuals who are likely to enjoy and benefit from this kind of activity.

Developmental groups that grow out of support groups such as women's groups, Parents Without Partners, or Alcoholics Anonymous tend to start with a small core of interested persons and to grow through networks set up for the support group as a whole. Bibliotherapy sessions may occasionally be scheduled as one facet of a training seminar, retreat, or encounter group. In such cases, recruiting is not separate from that done for the activity in general.

For all groups meant to be ongoing, the facilitator should plan one or two meetings or coffees to introduce the basic goals and procedures of bibliotherapy. Be sure to take down the names, addresses, and phone numbers of all potential members to facilitate the scheduling of personal interviews and group meetings.

Recruitment of participants in the school setting is often somewhat more formalized. Some English teachers have scheduled bibliotherapy as a regular part of their classroom activities. However, although many students will benefit from this exposure to literature as a vehicle for understanding themselves, the teacher must scrupulously avoid evaluating their participation as part of a grade.

In other cases, referrals to the bibliotherapy group come from the school counselor. Actual membership may be affected by the kind of arrangements that can be made for scheduling group sessions during the school day. At times, the librarian will take responsibility for scheduling and facilitating groups; at other times, an individual teacher or counselor will identify potential members and arrange the sessions. Counseling departments in colleges and universities may offer bibliotherapy as one form of group therapy in their mental-health support programs.

In still other cases, participants will come to bibliotherapy through professional referral or recruitment. For example, bibliotherapy may be one part of an established hospice program, or it might be offered in conjunction with other services for chronically ill or handicapped persons. Social workers dealing with battered women or unmarried teenagers, or in training programs themselves, have often made bibliotherapy part of their methodologies. Although such participants may have greater and more specific needs than those drawn to a public library group, these groups are considered to be developmental rather than clinical.

Screening

The initial screening and interviewing of potential participants for an open developmental bibliotherapy group can be more difficult to manage and may not be nearly as necessary as the screening of residents in an institution or of those seeking a therapeutic contact. In general, the purpose of the screening is to give the facilitator a better sense of the individual personalities, interests, and needs of the participants. At the same time, this one-on-one interchange can help future members get a better sense of the bibliotherapist as an empathic, trustworthy person.

As helpful as initial personal interviews can be, it is not always possible for a developmental bibliotherapist to arrange such meetings. In open groups established through a church, library, or common interest group, the most workable format may be to establish an introductory term of six to eight weeks and to agree that at the end of that time, the facilitator and the group will reevaluate whether or not to continue. At this point, the facilitator should have a sense of which individuals need to be referred for professional help or have other difficulties within the group. By the same token, some individuals will decide that they are not comfortable with the group and drop out at the end of the trial period.

Although the range of people who can benefit from developmental bibliotherapy is more inclusive than exclusive, there are cases in which the bibliotherapist will decide that an individual should not begin (or continue) with a developmental group. In the first place, developmental bibliotherapy can attract persons who are in need of a more intensive therapy. As we have indicated, the bibliotherapist who sees evidence of problems that cannot be dealt with adequately in the developmental setting is responsible for referring the people in question for more appropriate help. Clearly, in order to make such referrals, developmental bibliotherapists must familiarize themselves with local mental-health resources. They are also advised to include some training in a mental-health setting. Such exposure will increase the facilitator's capacity to recognize how deep-seated problems can be masked and will aid the delicate task of persuading a resistant individual to seek professional help.

In a few cases, it could be appropriate for an individual with a serious mental-health problem to remain in a developmental group. However, the facilitator must feel confident in such cases that the person's problems will not distort or interfere with the other group members' progress toward normal growth and development and that the individual is getting the necessary treatment elsewhere at the same time.

There is one distinct pattern of response that cripples an individual's ability to benefit from developmental bibliotherapy. Some persons who fear their emotions insist on intellectualizing instead of genuinely dealing with their feeling-responses. Thus they inevitably focus on the techniques or structure of the material to avoid looking at how the work touches on issues or feelings that trouble them. The bibliotherapist should make every effort to bring these individuals to a recognition of the avoidance implicit in concentrating on literary analysis in a bibliotherapy session, and should work to help them come to terms with emotion. But there will be cases in which one person's persistence in intellectualizing holds back the entire group. The facilitator may be forced to "counsel out" such an individual in order to allow other participants the full benefits of the bibliotherapeutic method.

The bibliotherapist depends on his or her professional judgment to decide whether or not to exclude a potential or currently participating group member because of needs that seem to extend outside the facilitator's therapeutic boundaries or because the individual seems strongly resistant to growing through bibliotherapy. In all such cases, the bibliotherapist initiates the discussion and makes the final decision. This is not a matter in which the group has a right to be involved.

Logistical Responsibilities

In addition to recruiting and screening members, the bibliotherapist is responsible for arranging such logistical details as timing and setting.

Timing

We have seen that the bibliotherapeutic process has a cumulative effect. Not only do participants grow in their ability to dialogue, but they often build on insights from the previous meeting or series of meetings as well. Thus the facilitator always arranges for meetings to be held at regularly scheduled intervals. Most groups meet weekly—a frequency that seems to be critical for clinical participants. Although some developmental groups will go two weeks between sessions, groups that try meeting once a month find that there is little continuity between sessions and that too much time is spent in reestablishing the proper climate.

In some cases, the interval between sessions is quite short. Developmental bibliotherapy sessions that are part of a workshop, retreat, or encounter weekend may be scheduled once a day or even each morning and afternoon for the days involved. Intensive programs, such as those designed for very acute patients or for short-term drug or alcohol abuse rehabilitation groups, may also ask the bibliotherapist to work with clients twice a week or even more frequently.

For either a clinical or a developmental group, the bibliotherapist is the person responsible for seeing that schedules are coordinated in such a way that a workable time (day and hour) is found for all group members. In an institutional setting, it is important to consult and consider other staff members in scheduling decisions so that they feel involved and are willing to cooperate with the bibliotherapy program. On the other hand, the scheduling for development groups tends to be more flexible. In either case, the timing should reflect the needs and makeup of the group.

Session length. Bibliotherapists working in institutions may have little choice about the length of time available for each session. Schools and universities are almost always restricted to forty- or fifty-minute periods; likewise, prisons and hospitals may be able to provide only for specified blocks of times for activities such as bibliotherapy. But when the facilitator has a choice, the length of time scheduled for each session depends largely on the attention span of the group members. A half-hour is likely to be enough for a group of regressed or very agitated mental patients. Similarly, young children, retarded persons, and hyperactive youths cannot be expected to attend for much longer than thirty or forty minutes at a time. However, the time span may be lengthened after several months when participants have become familiar with and involved in the bibliotherapeutic process.

At the other end of the scale, some developmental groups will be made up of very verbal participants who can easily sustain discussions of an hour and a half in length. However, even the most enthusiastic group should not go on for more than two hours, as there is an optimum time period during which effective stimulation can occur. As is true for most group activities, it is best to quit while you're ahead—when interest is high and before everything has been said. In that way, something is left over to be considered in the interval—some idea or issue that is ready to be sparked by the material in the next session. In general, then, the fifty-minute hour seems to be the most productive length for most groups.

Number of sessions. When either a clinical or a developmental bibliotherapy group is first established, an initial trial term should be set. At the end of six or eight weeks, both the bibliotherapist and the participants will have the option to terminate the group without undue embarrassment. In our experience, this option has seldom been exercised; however, we have found that the act of committing to further meetings at this point helps build cohesion.

Once the trial stage is passed, circumstances usually help determine how long a particular group will continue meeting. In some cases, a group might meet consistently at a given time and place for years, even though the actual population is likely to shift as some participants leave and others join. On the other hand, groups established through a school normally come to an end at the semester or year-end break. In other settings, the seasons of the year will provide convenient time divisions. Moreover, there will be times when the group and facilitator decide together that the group purpose has been achieved. Alternatively, the life circumstances of either the participants or the bibliotherapist can lead to the breaking up of the group. In Chapter 12, we will discuss the process of termination.

Setting

The bibliotherapist is responsible for determining where the bibliotherapy group will meet and for making any necessary arrangements, including the steps necessary to ensure that a sufficient number of chairs are available and set up. In many cases, the setting is determined by the nature of the group: Clinical groups will meet within the hospital; the church, synagogue, or community center sponsoring the group will have specified meeting rooms; and so on. But as the facilitator may still have some choice of the actual room to be used, he or she should make every attempt to keep the physical environment attractive and comfortable.

The libraries in institutions often provide an inviting setting with an established ambiance in which patrons sense both acceptance and the expectation that they will behave in a way that is acceptable to the world at large. In addition, lethargic and withdrawn patients often find that a group meeting scheduled in the library provides an incentive to leave the dormitory unit. At the same time, the magazines, newspapers, and books on display can stimulate a patient's awareness of the here and now.

On a very practical level, the decision to hold meetings in the library saves the bibliotherapist from logistical maneuvering. The books from which bibliotherapy materials are drawn are at hand both for facilitator and participants. In addition, most libraries have some facilities for using the audiovisual materials in their collection. Public libraries, too, offer the same comfortable atmosphere and ready access to materials. They are also typically open for extended hours, so that scheduling for meeting times is fairly flexible. For the most part, libraries are usually located in readily available places and already serve many sectors of the community.

Social Boundaries

Whether the bibliotherapy sessions are clinical or developmental, one-on-one or group oriented, it is the facilitator who is ultimately responsible for setting and maintaining the appropriate boundaries. Although the bibliotherapist makes the final decision about social—or procedural—policies, these issues should always be discussed and accepted by the group. In developmental groups in particular, decisions about mode of address, discussion methods, and general deportment are, in fact, group choices.

Mode of address

The decision as to whether it is more appropriate to use first or last names will vary from one group to the next. There are several factors to keep in mind when making the decision. Institutionalization is often both depersonalizing and humiliating. Patients and prisoners often have the impression that the institutional structure and personnel think of them as little more than numbers. A particular prisoner may grow tired of being brusquely addressed as "Jones," while a hospitalized depressive patient may resent the brisk "Well, Anna, how are we today?" from someone she is expected to respond to formally as "Doctor S." Thus, many clinical participants and prisoners seek the use of a formal mode of address (such as "Mr. McCue," "Miss March," etc.) as significant affirmation of the respect and dignity with which the facilitator regards them.

In other cases, the bibliotherapist recognizes social or cultural conventions that indicate whether a given group would be more comfortable with one mode over others. Clearly children might be confused if addressed as Mr. and Miss; older persons might interpret the use of first names as rude and presumptuous; whole subgroups of our culture consider formal address to be somewhat pretentious; and developmental groups open to general membership, or groups that have grown out of another support group or organization, may be made up of people who are already on a first-name basis.

The intake interviews may indicate what mode is likely to be appropriate for any given group. But if there is any uncertainty, it is always easier to move from more formal to less formal terms.

Interactions

Clinical bibliotherapists who have an explicit contract to provide therapeutic help will be more concerned with maintaining boundaries than will bibliotherapists working with developmental participants. In fact, in some developmental groups there is very little real difference between the facilitator and the participants. Such interchange of roles was very striking in a group of mental-health professionals who rotated responsibility for facilitating from session to session.

Those coming to bibliotherapy from a mental-health background will recognize that a certain amount of distancing is necessary in a productive therapeutic relationship. The clinical bibliotherapist must be alert to the various ways in which one or another participant in a group may try to establish a privileged relationship with the facilitator, such as by engaging in private therapeutic conversation outside the group meeting or by bringing gifts. The motivations behind such actions are many and varied. But the bibliotherapist must make it clear that he or she feels an equal responsibility to all group members and that there will be no special treatment or favoring of one over the others. In addition, all members of a group should be brought to see that an implicit or explicit contract has been made for *group* bibliotherapy and that all issues should be dealt with in that collective context. Sometimes it is enough for the bibliotherapist to pointedly defer discussion of an issue until it can be looked at by the group as a whole.

Note that we are talking here about a continued pattern of behavior. As we have indicated, private consultations are in order when the bibliotherapist recognizes that one person has a serious problem that cannot be dealt with adequately in the group setting or when someone is seeking referrals for help with a crisis.

In addition to the facilitator-participant relationship, the bibliotherapist must keep an eye on intragroup relationships. For example, experienced facilitators recognize that it is very common for group members to seek out special friends and/or to wield influence in the group as a whole. Whether or not one accepts Bion's (1961) theory that there is deep psychological significance in such "pairing," the facilitator is responsible for seeing that such interactions do not get out of hand. At the same time, group members should be made aware of the dynamics involved.

Comportment

At the first meeting of every bibliotherapy group, the bibliotherapist should facilitate a discussion about what will be expected in terms of participation and behavior. It should be made clear that everyone must contribute to—and will benefit from—a climate characterized by cohesion and mutual support. As the group continues to meet, the bibliotherapist is responsible for being aware of and moderating the verbal and nonverbal behaviors that arise. When it is necessary to set boundaries, the facilitator should be firm without being caustic, aggressive, or arbitrary. In other words, it should be clear from the facilitator's manner that he or she has too much respect for self and for others to allow excessive behavior that makes others uncomfortable or puts them in any danger.

At times, the facilitator will need to articulate the fact that one individual's inappropriate or disruptive conduct interferes with everyone else's ability to benefit from the session. In fact, since issues of comportment are often actually group issues, the best strategy may be to turn to the group for decision making about what boundaries are to be set and how they can be enforced. However, if the others are intimidated by the disruptive participant, the facilitator should take direct action to free the group from whatever disturbance is affecting the climate. In extreme cases, it may be necessary to exclude an individual.

The degree to which specific policies must be discussed or spelled out varies considerably. Most developmental groups do not have to be told that carrying on private conversations, interrupting or insulting the speaker, or abruptly leaving the group is inappropriate. The bibliotherapist may have to take a much more active role in maintaining boundaries in a clinical group, however. In some cases, the treatment team or the bibliotherapist may feel it is necessary to set rules for behavior at the beginning of a clinical group and then to regularly re-involve the participants in rule-setting.

Note that the setting of sexual boundaries calls for particular sensitivity. Trainees should expect help from a supervisor as they learn to recognize, evaluate, and initiate effective procedures to deal with this issue. For example, overt sexual advances or masturbation in the group must be dealt with as both an individual and a group problem: The participants must learn to expect and to conform to society's standards for sexual behavior. But more subtle instances of inappropriate attachment to other group members or to the facilitator must be recognized and dealt with when they affect the climate or the dynamics of the therapeutic interaction.

Other areas of behavior are less sensitive, but they, too, have an impact on the group climate. For example, policies about attendance may become an issue, particularly in clinical groups. When one person always shows up late, the dialogue at each meeting is interrupted as the newcomer settles in. In addition to being an attention-getting device that shows lack of respect for others, this pattern could indicate that the person is resisting the kind of self-examination encouraged by bibliotherapy. Thus, when someone fails to show up at the scheduled hour, even after the group jointly sets a policy that members should be on time, the facilitator may have to confront the resistance directly. In extremely persistent cases, it may be necessary to exclude the individual in question, at least temporarily.

Other persons may find it difficult to stay throughout the time scheduled for a clinical group. When the literature or dialogue begins to turn toward a painful subject, anxious persons may wish to flee. They may just get up and leave, or they may express the wish to go to the bathroom or to get a drink of water. In some volatile settings, the facilitator may have to set the arbitrary rule that an individual who leaves before the session is over is not to return until the next meeting. In other cases, the group can be invited to help establish a policy for dealing with such difficulties.

Some other behavior issues are not as clear-cut and may come up in almost any group. For example, eating, drinking, and smoking are all activities that are acceptable in themselves under most circumstances. But passing around food, pouring (or accidently upsetting) drinks, or offering another a cigarette or a light can interrupt a train of thought or distract from a feeling-response. Some persons, moreover, will divert their expressions of feeling into eating or smoking instead of talking.

On the other hand, sharing food and drink or smoking can be a valuable tool for developing social skills and awareness of others. Persons who are institutionalized often have restricted access to snacks and cigarettes and may interpret these items as a special sign of caring and trust. Thus a clinical bibliotherapist might decide that the symbolism involved in eating or drinking will be therapeutic for a particular group. In such cases, the bibliotherapist usually arranges for coffee and cookies, or some equivalent, just before or after the actual dialogue. But the reasons for sharing and the way it is done should be periodically reevaluated in a group discussion.

The decision as to whether or not smoking should be allowed is more difficult. Cigarettes can be very precious to prisoners; some heavy smokers find it hard to attend to anything else when their systems are craving a cigarette. On the other hand, many nonsmokers dislike the fumes while others are actually allergic to cigarettes. Local smoking ordinances will resolve the dilemma in some locations; other groups will have to work out a solution for themselves. For example, one group in a women's shelter decided that only two people could smoke at any one time.

Similarly, dress or posture may seem inconsequential issues but if either draws attention away from the purpose of bibliotherapy, the issue should be dealt with in the group. Pronounced slouching, lying on the floor, or sitting with bare feet on the table are all behaviors that could distract other participants or the facilitator from the dialogue. Such postures may also suggest extreme disinterest or disrespect so that no useful work can be accomplished until a change is made. In addition, some people will be offended by halter tops on women or bare chests on men. Note that attitude, posture, or dress can become an issue in a one-on-one relationship as well as in a group. In all such situations, the matter should be discussed openly, and both the participants and the facilitator should honor the decision reached through mutual agreement.

Therapeutic Boundaries

In addition to resolving and maintaining policies having to do with social interactions, the bibliotherapist is responsible for seeing that each discussion is appropriately focused and that confidentiality is observed.

Appropriate topics for discussion

Almost any subject matter can be included within the scope of a bibliotherapeutic dialogue—so long as the discussion is genuine and growth directed. As these conditions are often not met, however, the bibliotherapist must frequently assert appropriate therapeutic boundaries for the discussion. For example, as we have already noted, the facilitator should firmly and quickly redirect any discussion that begins to demean any participant, to avoid true self-understanding, or to feed an unhealthy pattern of response. Clearly, too, the bibliotherapist must never permit the group to concentrate on the problems of a member who is not present at the meeting.

Once again, the clinical bibliotherapist is more likely to have to work actively on therapeutic boundaries than is the developmental group leader. For example, it is rarely therapeutic to allow a mental patient to go on at length about delusions or themes persistently introduced by this individual. Of course the facilitator may not recognize the delusion or preoccupation the first time it is brought up. But as soon as it is clear that the person's response is not reality-oriented in relation to the material or dialogue, or that the remark is one the patient has made repeatedly in different circumstances, the facilitator should intervene and redirect the dialogue. At times, it will be enough to say, "Perhaps it is now time to let others share their reactions." In other cases, the facilitator may have to break bluntly into a stream of talk: "Others need time now to express themselves. Please be quiet."

In both developmental and clinical groups, the bibliotherapist will face those times in which a participant introduces a topic that does not seem relevant to the dialogue. In this case, the individual may be having trouble expressing an obscure connection to the dialogue. But if no meaningful link becomes apparent, the facilitator should intervene with a remark such as "Do any of you see how this issue relates to what the rest of us are discussing?" Even while refocusing the discussion, the bibliotherapist should look for clues as to whether the inappropriate response came from a misunderstanding of the material or dialogue or from resistance to confronting the themes or ideas that were under discussion.

Finally, in some instances, the speaker may be someone who consistently talks for the sake of talking, with little concern for relevance. As in the case of delusional speakers, the facilitator owes it to the group to cut off such responses quickly and firmly. Even so, we should note again that, as important as it is to keep the dialogue productive, it is equally critical that the facilitator does not fall into prejudging what a certain person will say. Rather, the empathic guide looks for nonverbal clues, such as a more alert posture, that would indicate the person is more in tune with the present moment and thus should be encouraged to speak.

Confidentiality

Participants in a bibliotherapy group will not feel comfortable sharing their feelings unless they feel sure that they can trust the facilitator and the other group members not to use what they have said against them and not to betray their confidences to others outside the meeting. It is vital that all participants realize that the facilitator is bound by a strong ethical code to maintain confidentiality about therapeutic matters. However, different settings have somewhat different conditions. Most hospitals using team-treatment programs assume that team members will share information that has therapeutic significance in the interest of developing more effective treatment. At the first meeting of a clinical group, the bibliotherapist should make the situation clear: "As your bibliotherapist, you know that I will be discussing your treatment plan with other members of the staff. I will also being making progress notes on your charts, which you are free to read. How do you feel about that?"

The facilitator's obligation to maintain confidentiality may become an issue when a bibliotherapy trainee records, videotapes, or takes notes during a session. Institutions or community health centers may have a form they ask members to sign indicating that they do not object to the use of such records as long as the records are used with scrupulous discretion. If no such form is available, it is wise to protect both the members' rights and your own by having everyone sign a permission slip of the following sort:

> I give my permission to use the contents of this series of bibliotherapy sessions and the results of any research made in any written or audiovisual form. This material is to be used only for informational, educational, and/or research purposes in the mental-health field. I understand that my name will never be used.
>
> NAME: ______________________ DATE: ________________

Most participants accept the necessity of signing such a form as a matter of routine, once the purpose of both the notes and the form has been explained. In one actual case, however, a member of a short-term alcoholic group refused to sign. The facilitator did not press the point but indicated that the individual could keep silent while the tape was being made. When the man did speak up during a recording, the facilitator pointed out that he had done so. If there had been any resistance, that section of the tape would have been erased. But in fact, the opposition disappeared by the end of the first session.

Yet confidentiality is not just a matter between the facilitator and the individual participants. All group members should be involved in setting a policy among themselves: Do members feel that what is said in the group should be discussed only with group members, or is it all right to carry on a discussion with others outside the group? Moreover, is the issue of confidentiality important to the members?

As we have seen with other boundary issues, each group must work out a policy with which the individuals involved are comfortable. For some, confidentiality is not a significant matter. Patients who have been institutionalized for a long time, for example, may not seem to care much one way or another. On the other hand, members of support groups may feel that they already share a spirit of mutual respect and that they can assume that others will not abuse their trust when they share matters of great intimacy.

But confidentiality is a primary concern for others. For example, paranoid individuals in clinical groups and adolescents in most settings are particularly sensitive about how much they reveal of themselves and very conservative about whom they are willing to trust. At the same time, persons in correctional institutions are very much aware that all therapeutic materials may be used as part of the court proceedings. Rubin (1977) feels that prisoners will not feel free to utilize the literature and dialogue genuinely and therapeutically unless the facilitator can assure the group members that strict confidentiality will be maintained. Until more evaluation and research has been done on this topic, each bibliotherapist will have to decide personally the conditions under which he or she might feel that material disclosed in a bibliotherapy session should be shared with other staff members.

In any event, whether working with an individual or with a group, clinically or developmentally, the bibliotherapist is responsible for bringing up the issue of confidentiality very early on. Since the ethical standards between therapist and client are well established, the major area of such discussion will concern the ways in which participants should handle the information disclosed in the course of a group session. If the issue is met with indifference at first, the bibliotherapist should bring it up again at a later time, when the sharing begins to reach some depth. Note that the bibliotherapist's responsibility here is to bring the issue to open discussion and to facilitate an agreement among the members; this is definitely not a situation in which the bibliotherapist should make the decision for the group.

STUDY GUIDE

1. Outline the initial steps and logistical details for which the bibliotherapist is responsible when starting a new bibliotherapy group.

2. Read and report on one of the following articles about boundary management and include a statement detailing how the techniques and strategies could apply specifically to bibliotherapy sessions (in a class situation, reports can be presented in a panel): (a) Berger and Rosenbaum (1967), on help-rejecting complainers; (b) De Rosis (1978, Chapter 8), on expressing hostility to family; (c) Hammond (1978), on the use of confrontation; (d)

Johnson and Johnson (1982, Chapter 8), on the use of power; (e) Yalom (1975, pages 283–313), on problem patients; (f) Singer (1975b), for an overview of boundary problems; (g) any chapter of interest in Egan (1975) or Fromm-Reichman (1950).

3. Discuss the differences you foresee between facilitating a bibliotherapy session and leading a group in a capacity already familiar to you (e.g., classroom, traditional therapy, discussion leader, etc.). You may want to consider Ponzo's (1974) account of how he had to adapt his practice to the realities of counseling in a new situation and identify the adjustments he made.

PRACTICUM

1. Using what you know about the bibliotherapist's responsibilities, formulate a contract for presentation to an actual group or one that you hope to work with. Address the issues of modality, timing and setting, social boundaries, and confidentiality.

2. Imagine two specific groups you might work with—one clinical and one developmental. Outline your expectations of the feelings the participants are likely to express about boundary issues. Include a description of one situation in which you feel different boundary decisions could affect the course of the dialogue. Be prepared to discuss your ideas with other students or with your supervisor.

FURTHER READINGS

Borriello (1976) describes the preliminaries necessary for setting up any therapeutic group in a hospital or institution. Egan's (1975) generalized text for "the skilled helper" offers detailed information on attitudes and skills. Yalom's (1975, 1983) works, the most widely used texts on group methods, detail the responsibilities involved in creating groups and selecting methods; his 1983 textbook deals specifically with in-patient groups. For other textbooks on group methods, see the readings in Chapter 13 of this book. Jourard (1964) discusses attitudes that can affect the ways in which facilitators carry out specific responsibilities. See pages 1–30 on self-disclosure, pages 66–75 on resistance, and pages 153–155 on authenticity.

9

Strategies for Facilitating a Bibliotherapy Session

A clinical bibliotherapist was working with a group of chronic mental patients who were being readied for a move to another unit, where they would be prepared for living again in the community. The therapist had placed two baskets on the table in the middle of the room. One held unshelled peas, the other beans. The therapist asked the members to come and take a handful of each in turn to shell or snip.

Not everyone knew what to do with either the peas or the beans. But group members were encouraged to help one another and did so. Thus there was some talking and even laughter as the task was completed.

The participants were then invited to eat the raw vegetables they had just fixed, if they wished to do so. Without too much direction from the facilitator, participants talked about their having performed these same tasks before their illness. Following a few minutes of reaction to this warm-up experience, the facilitator handed out copies of a selection from Eric Hoffer's "The Ordeal of Change" *on the theme, "No one really likes the new." She read aloud the brief sketch that describes how Hoffer had spent a winter picking peas in California. Then in June he had shifted to picking string beans and became very hesitant about doing something different. He concluded, "Even the change from peas to string beans had in it elements of fear."*

When she finished reading, the facilitator was quiet for a minute. She could see one or two participants looking back over their own copy of the passage; others just sat. The facilitator nodded encouragingly at one woman who looked like she might have something to say.

"I liked doing the peas better," the woman said slowly. "I was a little mixed up with the beans at first." The bibliotherapist nodded sympathetically and commented, "You found the change confusing." The woman

felt encouraged to continue, "I don't like it when I don't know just what is right to do."

Others began to talk; then one man said he really disagreed with most of the others. He liked doing the beans better; "besides," he said, "they always cook the peas here until they're too mushy."

The facilitator felt that the focus should be turned back to the literature. She said, "We don't all have to like eating the same things. But let's try to think more about how we feel about differences or changes. Maybe we can get some ideas from looking at the last line of our story again." She then asked the woman who had first spoken to read the line aloud and to share how she felt about it. Once again, other participants were encouraged to look at how they personally responded to the idea that even simple changes involved some fear.

The time scheduled for bibliotherapy was almost up. The facilitator closed the meeting by saying, "We have done some good work today. But I think we need to look even harder at the way we feel about making changes. You may want to read your copy of our selection during the week. Think about what you could say on the subject next time."

THE BIBLIOTHERAPIST IS FACED REPEATEDLY with strategic decisions about the best way to facilitate the therapeutic dialogue. In this chapter we will review these decisions as they occur in the course of a session.

Basic Model for Introducing Materials Chosen by the Bibliotherapist

In a typical interactive bibliotherapy group meeting, the facilitator and group members are seated in their chairs, which are arranged in a circle to encourage cohesion and interaction. When copies of the material to be used for the day have been passed around, the bibliotherapist reads the selection aloud clearly. The reading is followed by a moment of silence so that the impact of the piece can sink in. If the selection is short and especially pithy, or if the facilitator knows that the participants will rely on oral presentation rather than on looking at the text, the work may be read through a second time.

The discussion should begin with an open-ended remark. The comment can be totally nondirective: "Does anyone have anything to say now that we have heard the poem?" "Let us talk about the ideas in this piece," or "Well, that is the story. There were probably some things you liked about it and some things you did not." If the session has been planned around a theme that is an area of concern for most people in the group, the question can reflect that theme. "Does this piece suggest anything about friendship to you?"

We have seen how a theme can develop out of a series of sessions. In such cases, the initiating remark can reflect that continuity: "In discussing last week's selection, we talked about how it feels to face a new situation. What does this selection suggest to you about the feelings you experience when you try something new?"

The basic model for introducing the material is often modified by involving the participants directly in the presentation. After the first reading—or, in some cases, *for* the first reading—the facilitator can invite one or two of the members to read the material aloud or to read a line they find especially significant. When members are uneasy about their reading ability, the facilitator may decide to read first and then have the whole group join in on a *choral reading.*

Seating arrangements and the decision as to who should read the selection will be somewhat different in a one-on-one bibliotherapy session, but the therapist will decide among the same kind of initiating questions and remarks.

Modified Model for Use of Audiovisual Material

The basic model for presenting materials must be modified somewhat when audiovisuals are being used. In particular, the facilitator should use strategies that will prevent the mechanics of such use from interfering with the dialogue. For example, the projector or record player should already be set up when participants enter the room and the film or tape advanced to the starting place. The bibliotherapist can also invite group members to help arrange the seating so that everyone can see the screen and then, when the viewing is over, to move the chairs back into a circle.

When only a segment of a film, recording, or video is being used, the facilitator should simply but clearly explain what has happened up to the point at which the screening begins. In the absence of such a summary, spontaneous responses are often diffused as the participants try to figure out what is going on.

Modified Model for Use of Warm-ups and Complementary Material

Although the examples in the following discussion will be based on group sessions, warm-ups and complementary materials can be used in one-on-one interactive bibliotherapy as well.

Warm-ups

Warm-ups are especially effective for leading into (1) sessions early in the history of a group, (2) sessions with participants that are hard to stimulate, or (3) sessions in which the chosen topic treats a sensitive issue. As the term itself indicates, warm-ups are not meant to become the focus of the entire session but, rather, are intended to help the participants feel freer and more comfortable with responding on a personal level.

Thus, early in the history of the group, the bibliotherapist might decide to open each session with a simple exchange that will help group members become aware of each other as individuals, such as having participants share their names and one statement about themselves. At other times, the group might begin by having members state their favorite color or what time of year they like best.

Other warm-ups can be used at any point in the history of the group to help the participants move from other routines into an open, reflective frame of mind. For example, Clancy and Lauer (1978) suggest the use of Zen telegrams, whereby the facilitator sees that each participant has a paint brush, ink, and a piece of white paper. Members are asked to close their eyes and create some brush strokes. The facilitator then asks everyone to look at what they have done and to tell the group in a word or phrase how their drawing makes them feel. The nonjudgmental experimentation and spontaneous choice of words that characterize this activity seems to help free members to respond to whatever the facilitator has planned for the main focus of the session (Reps 1959).

Visual complementary material

A warm-up can be tailored to lead directly into the material for a given session. In many cases, it will involve some kind of *visual complement* to the material. For example, the facilitator might pass around a cartoon that will be a good lead-in to the themes found in a work selected for a developmental group session. Or clinical participants might be asked to look through magazines for a picture of a door that appeals to them before discussing David Antin's poem, "Doors." Then, one by one, members would be invited to hold up the picture they selected and tell something of what they felt in making the choice. Such warm-ups are particularly good for those who have trouble concentrating for long periods of time. They allow the participants to move into the topic in a totally personal but nonthreatening way and dispose them to continue making personal responses as the actual material is presented and discussed.

Joy Sheiman (1972), a California poetry therapist, has found many uses for her collection of pictures of masks. For example, participants can look for a mask that says something about themselves or shows what they do or do not want to be. This exercise could be a warm-up either for a specific selection to be read aloud or for a creative writing assignment.

Clearly many different warm-up techniques are possible. Some have been described in examples throughout this book. In the next chapter we will detail other techniques specifically designed to loosen members up to do original writing. Schloss lists a variety of warm-ups in his essay in Lerner's book (1978). In addition, Ballard's (1982) manual for group leaders includes a variety of excellent techniques and ideas that are readily adaptable. Assignments designed to extend student reading and writing might also be used to good advantage.

As trainees gain experience, they will develop their own catalogue of techniques. It is worth the trouble to develop a file of warm-ups that have proved to be especially effective. The activity should be cross-referenced on the use record kept in the author card file. Regardless of the technique used, however, it is important to recognize that an activity meant as a warm-up may put a participant in touch with highly significant personal feelings. The facilitator will need skill and perception to take advantage of such moments. The most effective strategy may be to deal immediately and in depth with the issue that has been raised. Or perhaps the material included as the primary focus of the dialogue can be used to explode the flash of self-understanding generated by the warm-up into a real understanding. The facilitator will have to decide which approach best answers the needs of a given case and, once again, will have to be flexible enough to shift the planned direction of the meeting if necessary. On the whole, however, warm-ups remain just that—freeing experiences that open members up to opening themselves to exploring genuine feeling-responses.

Realia as complementary material

The bibliotherapist can also introduce a selection by having the participants interact in some way with a real object that is related to the idea or situation described in the material. For instance, participants might try on hats, finger the luxurious texture of velvet slippers, pick out a stone or a seashell whose texture or design particularly appeals to them, handle the jumping ropes and jacks of childhood games, or enjoy the special smell and taste of fresh bread. The use of such *realia* (the term is taken from the education field) involves the participants' sensory perceptions in such a way that they tend to respond more strongly and immediately to the images and objects that are presented directly afterward in the primary bibliotherapeutic material. Again, as we saw in the opening vignette, a feeling-response can actually be sparked by the complementary object or activity and then focused by the material and the dialogue.

Handicapped people will appreciate this appeal to more than one sense; children, senior citizens, and special-education groups may also find that contact with a concrete object makes it easier to bring imaginative material to life. Chronic and regressed patients can be very reluctant to move, but when asked to come to a coffee table to handle materials, they may well have some motivation for breaking out of their usual pattern of passive withdrawal.

In one case, after several weeks of bibliotherapy sessions in which the material was introduced with realia, the facilitator found that the participants in the chronic ward were talking to each other, learning each other's names, handing items on without being asked, and even picking up fallen things to hand them to the owner. Although such gestures may seem perfectly normal to those who do not have problems with socialization, this kind of interaction was a significant step in breaking down the isolation and dulling of responses that affects many who are institutionalized.

As important as it is to enhance the clinical patient's capacity to respond in a fundamental way, developmental participants of all types also find that their responses are enhanced by the strategic use of realia. Even familiar objects can take on a new meaning when handled in the context of a bibliotherapy session. There is increasing evidence that the more completely one is engaged in a healthy response, the more beneficial it is likely to be. So, although bibliotherapists should not try to duplicate what happens in music, dance, art, or drama therapy, they can incorporate some of the techniques and insights that come from these fields. Bibliotherapists should regularly check for ideas and discussions listed under the topic heading of *sensory perception* in mental-health indexes.

Nonetheless, as enriching as it can be to use realia to introduce the primary bibliotherapy material, this strategy should be used thoughtfully. Here, again, the facilitator must depend on intuition, training, and experience to judge the actual effect a particular object or activity might have on a given group. Moreover, as we saw in our discussion of the strategic choice of material, something that answers the needs of a group in one situation might be unsatisfactory in a different context.

Auditory complementary material

In some cases, a work is better enhanced by an auditory complement than by realia. For example, song lyrics can be presented with musical accompaniment, or instrumental music can act as an effective backdrop for a filmstrip or for a reading. In other cases, the music can precede or follow the actual chosen material. For example, "mood music" can help set the tone for the material to follow or to stimulate a creative writing exercise. One facilitator found that she could start focusing the attention of a very restless group when she signaled the opening of the group by playing arresting, unfamiliar ethnic rhythms such as Japanese Noh music or songs played on the Indian zither. (Folkway Records has an excellent selection of such works.)

But auditory complements need not always be music as such. With the use of special-effects tapes and records, the sounds of the wind, the rain, the sea, or a crackling fire can add to the intensity of a particular work.

Alternatively, the bibliotherapist might decide that it would be effective to have the participants make music of their own—either through rhythmic clapping, humming, and singing, or by using simple instruments provided by the bibliotherapist. The complementary activity should not overshadow the dialogue, of course, but we have found nonetheless that sound and music can significantly enhance the impact of bibliotherapeutic material.

Complementary art material

In addition to their use as warm-ups, art materials can be employed effectively to initiate the bibliotherapeutic process *after* the literature has been presented. In this procedure, participants are provided with large sheets of paper, felt-tip pens, crayons, paints, or modeling clay and asked to visually express their responses to what they have just heard. Those who protest that they can't draw will be helped to see that no judgments will be made about the results. Frequently, those who are most intimidated end up delighted with this form of expression—once they feel free to use it. Note that, in some cases, the participants respond more successfully when the bibliotherapist joins in the activity; in other cases, individuals may be intimidated and discouraged by the apparent ease with which the facilitator is working. The bibliotherapist will have to make a strategic decision as to what strategy is best for each circumstance. Of course, although everyone should be encouraged, no one should be forced into participating. (See Mitchell 1978 for a description of the different variations she has used to combine painting and poetry in a mental hospital.)

In bibliotherapy, the art activity is not an end in itself. All participants will be asked to express something about their pictures and will be helped to examine the insights triggered by the combination of the material and their own visual expressions of response.

Overview of strategies for presenting material

There are many instances in which a facilitator will decide that it is more advantageous to introduce the literature for a given session by using the text alone. Complementary material is meant to stimulate response, not to dominate the literature and its message. The latter may happen when group members come to expect this kind of lead-in and thus lose their capacity to respond spontaneously to the work itself. On the other hand, the use of realia or other complements can be somewhat directive; that is, the complement may draw attention to the aspect of the material that relates to the concrete object or activity. In doing so, however, the complements can leave a participant a little less free to recognize something in the piece that is uniquely meaningful. Finally, the bibliotherapist who depends heavily on realia or auditory or visual complements to introduce the literature will find that the strategy both limits the choice of potential material and cuts into the amount of time available for the dialogue.

Selections Made by Participants

Given the life circumstances of the participants, or logistical considerations in general, it is often most practical and effective to ask bibliotherapy participants to spend some of the meeting time in choosing a poem or work to share with the group. When the selection is to be made in the group setting, the facilitator must bring in an adequate number of anthologies, textbooks, or loose copies of poems taken from the files. The materials should be spread out so that members can easily browse through them. The members should also be given some direction. Sometimes the invitation is quite general: "Look for a poem that you like," or "Find a poem that says something you would like to share with the group." At other times, particularly when the group is focusing on a particular theme or issue, appropriate selections can be culled from the file and duplicated for use.

In either situation, the facilitator should allow enough time to give most participants a chance to make a comfortable choice. Inevitably, some will seem to pick the first item that they look at, whereas others will be in agony trying to find the perfect piece. The facilitator should make it clear that no judgments are being made about the individual based on the style in which the choice is made. Our experience has been that even the clinical patients who seemed to have made their choices hastily and at random are able to express at least something they find personally meaningful in the selection when they begin to discuss it.

The bibliotherapist is responsible for deciding how the selections are to be presented and discussed. In some cases, the decision will be to leave the logistics to the will of the group. Developmental groups often seem to run themselves, for example. At other times, the facilitator will draw on the knowledge of the individual members and on his or her experience with the group to decide on the order in which presentations should be made and on who will do the reading.

Although all members should be encouraged to share their selections, the principle of noncoercion applies once again. That is, if an individual expresses or indicates unwillingness to participate, the facilitator should move calmly on to the next person. At the same time, however, the facilitator must be alert for nonverbal indications as to whether the resistance is deep-seated or can be overcome. Sometimes a participant who declined to share at first will feel freed to do so after observing the presentation and discussion of several other pieces. The facilitator may quietly offer the reluctant person another chance after the other selections have been gone through; every so often, that person may even volunteer to share.

A sensitive bibliotherapist recognizes that a self-belittling remark such as "Mine isn't very good" or "Probably no one will like the poem I choose" often masks a cry of insecurity and/or may be a plea for extra attention. In either case, it is not really helpful to feed this kind of manipulation with effusive protests and reassurances. Rather, experienced facilitators often find quiet, matter-of-fact affirmations to be more effective: "You made a choice that means something to you; that's what makes it good. We would like you to share your selection now."

The actual reading aloud of a selected poem may be done by the individual participants. Once the selections have been made, individual participants may volunteer or respond to an invitation to present their selections to the group. However, it is important that the reading be done so that all present can hear and understand, as other participants will not have a text to which they can refer. Consequently, the facilitator may decide to do the reading when it becomes evident that several members will have difficulty with the oral presentation. In other instances, each person might be invited to share his or her selection with a remark such as this: "It is your turn now, Mr. X. Would you like to read the poem you have chosen, or would you prefer to have me present it?" On the other hand, a participant may ask another group member who is known as a good reader to read his or her selection. Again, the specific circumstances will influence the bibliotherapist's decision as to which strategy is most appropriate.

As each selection is presented, the bibliotherapist should offer some kind of respectful recognition of the individual's contribution. It can be a significant act for withdrawn participants simply to make and announce a choice; moreover, the facilitator might determine that recognition of this achievement is sufficient without probing into what motivated the choice. In other cases, the individual can be encouraged to explore the reasons for which a particular work seemed meaningful. Alternatively, it may be more productive to open the dialogue to other group members' feeling-responses to the choice.

There is no hard and fast rule as to how much time should be spent on any single selection; the facilitator will have to base that decision on the immediate circumstances. In most cases, however, the bibliotherapist should plan to spend more than one session going through the participants' selections, particularly when the group is large.

Note, too, that the use of participants' choices as material can affect the group atmosphere and/or bring up situations that call for active facilitation. For example, clinical participants can show surprisingly possessive feelings about the item they select to the extent that they are unable to distance themselves enough to discuss it; in other cases, an individual may be unwilling to have others comment on the selection. Still other participants will need to be reassured that moving on to another selection does not involve any rejection or belittling of the piece that has just been discussed.

It may also happen that one person's choice will strike another as artificial, threatening, or distasteful. So, too, some individuals will be fairly inarticulate or actually boring as they present or explain their selections. In fact, some choices will strike the facilitator personally as inappropriate, trite, or even insincerely made. The facilitator's role in all such cases is to be both genuine and respectful and to see that a therapeutic group atmosphere is maintained. Inexperienced persons can use supervisory help in sorting out when it is appropriate to prompt someone who is having difficulty, when someone should be cut off, and when the group should be involved in discussing the dynamics of the situation.

Selections Made Outside the Group

Although the bibliotherapeutic material is most often chosen by the facilitator or by participants in the group setting, there are times when it is very effective to have the participants select material between sessions. In fact, developmental groups organized through a library or support group may establish a policy of having group members systematically share responsibility for the material. This strategy can be problematic with many clinical groups, but some—such as chemical dependency groups—benefit greatly from being asked occasionally to take more time than is available in the course of a session to pick out a work that is personally meaningful.

The strategies available for facilitating the sharing by each member of his or her choice are similar to those used when the material is selected within the group setting. However, the time lapse between choice and presentation may make it more practical to duplicate the work so that each member will have a copy of the text to refer to in the dialogue. Once again, the bibliotherapist depends on sensitivity, experience, and training to determine when to move from one selection to the next.

Furthermore, as the selections were made in a context that allowed more time for reflection than is possible in a single session, it can be fruitful to direct the dialogue toward an examination of what went on in the process. The facilitator might open discussion of a selection by asking participants what emotions or considerations came to mind as they went through the selection process; alternatively, the dialogue might explore exactly what made the item seem a good choice. Note that the time lapse between the selection and actual presentation of a piece can in itself be revealing. As it is discussed in the group setting, the item may take on a meaning or force that the participant missed when the original selection was made. In such cases, a good bibliotherapist is prepared to help the individual look more closely to see if there is anything significant in the way his or her perspective has changed.

On occasion, an individual in a developmental or clinical group will spontaneously volunteer to share a selection with the group. The bibliotherapist must always be respectful of such overtures and may agree to use the selection in a future meeting or at the end of the current session. However, not every such offering will be appropriate or beneficial for the group as a whole, and the facilitator must be prepared to clearly and respectfully explain that situation as well.

Even if the facilitator is not choosing the material for a session, it is still his or her responsibility to make sure that all group members know in advance if they are to bring in material for a future session. The bibliotherapist should also have a back-up item in reserve in case there is some mix-up or lapse.

Interventions in the Dialogue

Up to this point, the chapter has concentrated on initiating strategies—that is, on the different ways in which material can be introduced. Now we can review the kinds of interventions used to facilitate the bibliotherapeutic dialogue. But, first, let us once again note the basic assumption that should inform all strategic decisions about activities or dialogue: *The literature is a tool for therapeutic discussion; hence the focus is always on the personal feeling-response and not on the meaning of the material itself.*

One corollary of this assumption is that all facilitative interventions will be designed to involve members in personal opinions and personal experiences rather than to objectively explore theoretical or intellectual issues. Thus the bibliotherapist typically uses personal pronouns such as "you," "your," "I," and "ours" in facilitating remarks rather than asking what the author meant or how an impersonal "they" might respond or even why "they" or "he" might feel as they do.

A second corollary of the assumption is that the purpose of the discussion is not to produce a consensus or a common understanding of the material but to further each person's unique understanding of his or her self. Thus the bibliotherapist must encourage and manage diversity but must do so in a way that creates a climate of mutual respect and support among group members.

Skilled intervention is the key to good bibliotherapy. Whether evaluating one's own performance or supervising another, the same two criteria are used: (1) Was the intervention of a sort that is appropriate to bibliotherapy? And (2), was the intervention strategically advantageous in the specific circumstances, or might another sort of approach have been more effective?

Both of these standards should be kept in mind throughout the following survey of the major kind of bibliotherapeutic interventions. Note that this outline is meant to be suggestive rather than exhaustive. Serious students of bibliotherapy will do more reading in the many texts devoted to therapeutic techniques with groups and individuals.

Nondirective invitations to respond

In the interest of keeping the dialogue as open as possible, many facilitating remarks are nondirective. We have seen, for example, that initiating remarks are often open-ended: "How did you feel as you heard this poem?" "Is there anyone who would like to share his reaction to this story?" It may also be advantageous to ask a nondirective question when a member makes an observation or reveals a memory that the facilitator feels is worth probing: "Would you like to tell us more about what you just said?"

Of course, some persons do need to be given some direction. Thus bibliotherapists will often focus on a particular moment in the literature in an open-ended way. For example, in Dorothy Canfield Fisher's story "The Heyday of the Blood," an adult remembers a childhood excursion with his grandfather and reflects on the grandfather's motto, "Live while you live, and then die and be done with it." A bibliotherapist might ask, "What is your personal response to the grandfather's motto?" This phrasing leaves participants free to respond with a whole spectrum of reactions from passionate agreement with such a philosophy, to indifference, to vehement opposition. The wording also allows participants to orient the dialogue in different ways. One person might answer by saying "My grandfather would never have said that. He always wanted my parents and me to plan for the future." This response might turn the discussion to a consideration of family relationships rather than the value of the motto.

There is a real art to posing truly open-ended questions. Exact phrasing can be crucial. It may seem that there is little difference between the question just given and asking "Is the grandfather's motto a good one?" But this second version is directive in a way that tends to undercut the bibliotherapeutic dialogue. In the first place, "good" implies a judgmental response. At the same time, the phrasing removes emphasis from a personal reaction; that is, the discussion could easily drift into the subject of whether people in general could or should live according to such a principle. Finally, a participant could answer with a simple "yes" or "no" or "it's all right" rather than use the intervention to examine his or her personal response.

Note, too, that nondirective facilitations are not always phrased as questions. Bibliotherapists frequently use *affirming statements of encourage-*

ment such as, "Yes, I see what you are saying," or "That seems to be something you feel strongly." This kind of remark shows the participant who is struggling to express something that he or she is being heard and that the effort is worthwhile and should be continued.

At times, the affirmation may take the form of *active listening*. The therapist restates—without interpreting or judging—what the participant has just said. "You mean your grandfather wanted you and your parents to think about the future rather than 'live while you live' as the motto in the story suggested?" As the participant assesses the accuracy of the restatement, he or she may also be brought to productive questioning of whether the original statement does express what the individual actually feels or means.

In short, nondirective facilitations implicitly communicate the therapist's empathy, respect, and confidence in the individual participants. Not only are such interventions nonjudgmental, but they also assume that the group members can discover for themselves something that is uniquely meaningful in the literature.

Nonverbal facilitations

The facilitator must accurately interpret the nonverbal expressions of the group members, but it is equally crucial that he or she use nonverbals effectively and strategically. As we have already noted, many people are intuitively sensitive to the respect and acceptance that can be communicated through the bibliotherapist's bearing and attitude. Moreover, the facilitator will find that there are many occasions in which the most effective nondirective affirmation or encouragement is a nod, a murmur of approval or sympathy, a smile, or a gesture.

Perhaps the most powerful item in the bibliotherapist's nonverbal vocabulary is *silence*. But strategic silence is also one of the most difficult techniques to learn to use effectively. Beginning trainees regularly struggle with the panic-stricken assumption that any lapse in the discussion is a strained silence that should be filled. Through experience and supervision, however, they learn to recognize and use *productive silence*. We have seen how experienced bibliotherapists regularly allow a few moments of reflection just after the bibliotherapeutic material is presented. Depending on the group, this silence may be broken by some kind of facilitating remark, or by a spontaneous response from one of the members. So, too, there will be times in the course of a dialogue when the group as a whole or one individual is absorbed in mentally working on an issue. The facilitator learns to recognize those times when an insight might be lost because the person was pressed to verbalize too soon. In other cases, an individual will find it easier to respond to expectant silence than to articulate some complex reaction in answer to a specific question.

Bibliotherapists also learn the value of *empathic silence.* Both the facilitator and other group members may find quiet sympathy to be the best acknowledgment of a deeply felt statement or a painfully won insight. Of course, empathic silence may be accompanied by other nonverbals such as a nod, a murmur, or, if appropriate, a light touch.

Directive facilitations

As valuable as nondirective interventions can be, there are many points at which the bibliotherapist must ask questions or make remarks that explicitly direct the dialogue: Sometimes the facilitator must help an individual or the group as a whole to focus scattered responses in some coherent way; at other times, a specific resistance must be dealt with and overcome before healing and growth can take place. But even more often, developmental and clinical participants alike simply are not accustomed to being precise about what they feel and think or how they understand a connection between the literature or dialogue and their experience. In such cases as these, facilitating questions and remarks can help them reach their inner selves.

Trainees in particular should make it part of their preparation to think through questions and remarks that could be used when the dialogue falters. Although many of these interventions will not be used, at least the bibliotherapist will be prepared to effectively facilitate the dialogue out of an unresponsive silence instead of reacting with panic.

The kinds of interventions that provide specific direction vary widely:

1. The remark may focus on an issue but leave the approach fairly open: "Many of you have been expressing uneasiness about the idea that you sometimes have to depend on other people. Let's talk about that."

2. The facilitation will work on drawing out a response: "That line of poetry seemed to remind you of something specific. Can you tell us about it?" Or "Your reaction to Mr. X.'s experience seems very strong. Perhaps something like that happened to you. We want to give you some time to think about it and tell us about it."

3. Sometimes it is important to bring out specific details: "You said that the story reminded you of a camping trip you took as a child. Exactly what was it about the experience or characters that seemed familiar?" Or "Tell us in more detail what you did and felt just before you lost your temper."

4. Discrepancies may indicate important issues that need to be looked at more closely: "It seems to me that you are saying something a bit different from what I thought I heard a few minutes ago. Can you clarify?" Or "You have been expressing how you felt just after this incident. But I get the impression you no longer feel that way. Can you tell us something about how you feel now?"

5. The bibliotherapist may feel that a participant should be reinforced or directed toward an awareness of a personal strength: "It sounds as if you were really trying to decide what was best for your son." Or "You have begun to be much more open and honest about your feelings. All of us are learning something we can use for ourselves from what you are saying."

6. Directive remarks are also useful in facilitating intragroup dialogue. "Mr. B. just gave his opinion; does anyone else agree or disagree?" "Does anyone else want to comment?" Or "Miss Z.'s remark seems to be quite different from what you said a few minutes ago, Mr. J. Would you like to comment?"

7. Finally, as we saw in Chapter 8, concerning the bibliotherapist's responsibilities, the facilitator may have to intervene directly to work out issues involving inappropriate behavior, boundaries, or procedural items. Again, the bibliotherapist calls on both training and experience in deciding precisely how the intervention should be made. Very often the facilitator will have only a few minutes at most to weigh and decide on a strategy that takes into proper account the nature of the situation, the needs of the participant, and the legitimate rights of the other group members.

In one group, a participant refused to allow any discussion of Beatrice de Regniers's poem "I Looked in the Mirror." He declared that the poem was silly with such aggressive force that the other members were intimidated and fell silent. Thus the bibliotherapist had to draw on his skill and previous experience to determine what was behind such an adamant refusal and what would be the best course to follow, given the character of the protester and the needs of the other group members. One strategy would have been to substitute another piece so that the session could proceed. The facilitator would then have had more time to consider what personal issues the refusal was masking and how they could best be examined.

In this case, however, the bibliotherapist felt it was best for all concerned if the dialogue continued on the same work. But he also realized that he would have to turn the group around at this point and, in effect, begin again. So he first expressed his empathy, patience, and firmness with a remark to the objector: "Mr. Butler, we know how you feel about this poem. You think it has no value. Will you let us go on and talk about it anyway?"

If Mr. Butler had still refused to let the dialogue continue, the facilitator would have pointed out that expressing an opinion too vehemently means that others cannot exchange their thoughts and feelings. If that, and nothing else, had worked, the facilitator would have found it necessary to exclude the man.

To get the discussion going again after this interruption, the bibliotherapist re-presented the material. As he felt it was important to engage the participants as much as possible, he had the group as a whole read the poem aloud together. He then drew attention to some of its rather absurd images to lighten the tone and relax the group.

Characteristics of directive facilitations

Before we go on to the next type of intervention, let us summarize some of the features that are characteristic of good directive facilitations. As was true for nondirective interventions, the facilitator can direct the dialogue with statements as well as with actual questions. When someone needs encouragement or guidance but is willing and able to explore a critical issue, it can be advantageous to use statements such as some of those just given—statements that imply a question or direction but leave the initiative with the participant. In any case, however, both questions and statements should be *open-ended*. That is, if participants are not allowed to settle for a generalized response or a simple "yes" or "no," they can begin to genuinely probe their own reactions.

However, it takes time to get participants used to specifying and detailing their responses. The bibliotherapist may have to repeatedly and explicitly encourage individuals who are unwilling to look closely at their problem areas to be more precise and genuine. At the same time, it is important to remember that many of those in both clinical and developmental settings who find it difficult to articulate precisely what they feel or think are not hiding from deep-seated problems; they are simply not accustomed to acknowledging their feelings. Such participants may need explicit guidance for some time before they begin to take into account the important role that emotion plays even in normal patterns of response and of behavior.

In this regard, we should also note that good interventions usually do not begin with questioning *why* individuals feel as they do. That issue is almost always too diffuse and too complex to start with. But as you explore the exact what, where, how, when, and who questions related to an issue, the why often begins to emerge. In addition, whenever feasible, preface negative interventions with an empathic observation: "I can see that you would like to say more. But other people in the group also want to talk. Perhaps you will learn something different about how you yourself feel as you listen to their reactions." Or "The event you just told us about seems to make you feel very frustrated. Sometimes planning an action helps ease the frustration. But you have to get at why the action would help. Do you have any ideas?" Remarks that communicate empathic understanding not only make it easier for most people to express themselves; they also articulate why the individual will benefit from exploring the issue or conforming to the behavior.

Redirecting the focus of the dialogue

At least once or twice in the course of every bibliotherapy session the facilitator should intervene to change the focus of the dialogue. Some of these interventions can be anticipated. Thus the bibliotherapist will prepare some transition from the warm-up activity to the material, or from the material to the dialogue. By the same token, the facilitator will consider beforehand how to introduce any activity or writing assignment that he or she intends to use to wrap-up a meeting.

In addition, it is quite normal for the discussion to shift focus in the course of a session. As the discussion is proceeding, the facilitator may occasionally decide that it would be useful to explore an issue suggested by a remark or series of remarks in the dialogue or to pause to help one individual work on a critical area. Some shifts of this sort take place naturally; at other times, the facilitator will explicitly indicate that the dialogue is being refocused with a remark such as, "As we have been talking about what walls mean to you, several of you have mentioned how you feel about restrictions that are imposed by other people. Let us look at this question for a few minutes."

In other cases, the facilitator may see that some refocusing is absolutely necessary because the particular train of thought is not stimulating productive dialogue or because a given issue has been exhausted. Or the discussion may get stuck as one individual or group pursues an unhealthy focus. At such points the facilitator must decide which of several strategies best suits the circumstances and will then let the group know what is happening with either a nondirective or a directive intervention.

For example, the facilitator might say, "No one seems to have much to say. If we think about this other line of the poem, something new may appear." Alternatively, the facilitator might ask either one member or the group as a whole to read the whole piece, or invite members to pick one line or image that seems meaningful. In general, we have found that by going back to the text after some discussion we can trigger a fresh response and insight.

If the discussion flags, the bibliotherapist can turn to other questions or approaches that he or she thought of while preparing for the meeting. Or, if the group is usually very responsive, the facilitator might turn to the members for a new direction. "No one seems to be very involved with what we have said so far. Can one of you suggest something else you see in this poem that we could look at?"

Finally, at those times in which the chosen material absolutely falls flat or when the group is very restless or withdrawn, the bibliotherapist can decide to radically change strategies either by initiating a different activity, such as creative writing, or by introducing a second "back-up" piece. Note that both of these strategies may be either planned or resorted to as a means of salvaging the dialogue.

To a certain extent, a question of style is involved. Some bibliotherapists regularly plan to use both warm-ups and other primary materials and perhaps end with some writing as well. Others find it best to concentrate on one material or activity. Clearly, the bibliotherapist should take into account not only the character of each group but his or her own personal style as well.

The bibliotherapist must constantly weigh the advantages of offering direction against those of letting the participants do their own work. Clearly, every session is unique and no sure rules can be given. Trainees, for instance, tend to be more directive and to refocus the dialogue more often. Experienced bibliotherapists, on the other hand, have generally learned that each meeting tends to follow a certain discernible pattern. Even when the dialogue begins with a strong move forward, the issues may appear, later on, to have been exhausted. Whereas a trainee may feel obliged to revitalize the session by introducing a change, the experienced facilitator might see that this lull does not mean that everything has stopped. Often one participant or another spontaneously voices something new, at which point the dialogue will pick up again; then, suddenly, the first issue will reemerge in a more profound form. In other words, it is not always necessary to articulate the connections or to prod the change; sometimes it is only necessary to wait.

Closure

Just as the bibliotherapist is responsible for opening each session, it is his or her job to see that there is some closure for each meeting. In bibliotherapy, as in other therapeutic modes, only rarely will a session be allowed to continue for longer than the scheduled time. The process of understanding oneself is a continuous one. But it is not possible or productive to focus continuously and directly on that activity alone. Experience has shown that it is best to hold to a prearranged time frame.

We have noted that the facilitator is the time-keeper for a bibliotherapy session. But members frequently seem to have a built-in sense of timing; they often begin to sense the need to wind up as the session nears the end of the scheduled hour.

Decisions about the amount of time and the exact strategy to use to bring a given bibliotherapy meeting to a close are based on the nature of the individual group and members as well as on the way the meeting has gone. Some thought should be given to this matter as the facilitator prepares for the group session. But, here again, as we have seen, the facilitator must be flexible.

1. Closure may be signaled by a *summary* of the session, in which the facilitator sums up the meeting in a few sentences. Alternatively, one or

more members can be asked to assess what happened in the discussion. But it is important to remember that in many successful bibliotherapy meetings the members do not reach a consensus. The summary, therefore, may simply be a review of the issues touched on in the dialogue: "Today Robert Frost's poem helped us to see different ways to look at walls. Some of us talked about the kinds of fences we have built to keep other people out of our lives. Others worked on ways to use walls or boundaries in a productive way."

2. Just as a consensus is not always reached, bibliotherapy sessions do not always end with a resolution of the problematic issue. Both the facilitator and the members should realize that it is natural and fundamentally healthy to feel that some difficult aspect of human relationships or self-understanding still needs work. In such a situation, closure may consist of a brief recognition of the fact that the issue is not closed: "Today our discussion of this poem showed that we all still have much to learn about how we feel and how we plan to deal with loneliness."

3. Sometimes the facilitator will feel that the unresolved theme can still be productively explored by the group. Closure, in that instance, might consist of some expression of anticipation: "We have done some good work today on the problems we all experience when dealing with change. I will look for a piece to use next week that might give us another way to look at this issue." Alternatively, the facilitator could announce that the group will deal with the issue through another strategy, such as creative writing.

4. In still other situations, the meeting will be brought to a close through different forms of summary and anticipation. A bibliotherapist who senses that the group is no longer engaging in productive dialogue about a theme might announce that "we have spent some time and done some good work on the idea of loneliness. But we don't seem to be saying much new at this point. Therefore, next week we will look at another issue."

5. On the other hand, something already touched on peripherally may constitute an effective new focus, in which case the facilitator could include that possibility in the closing statement. Finally, the facilitator might either announce that the material for the following session will be a film or ask the participants to bring in a poem or a piece of creative writing for the next meeting.

6. We have said that literature is the primary tool of bibliotherapy. At times, the facilitator will close simply by *letting that tool continue its work:* "I see that our time is about up. We have touched on many different points today. But now I'd like to look at the poem again. Will you please join me in reading it aloud together? As we read, think of what today's discussion has meant to you."

7. As related strategies, the facilitator might read alone, ask someone who has responded in a special way to read, replay a recording or short film, or ask each participant to choose and read one line from the material that now seems especially significant.

8. Some bibliotherapists like to use wrap-up materials or activities. For instance, in the last few minutes of a session, members might be asked to reflect on the dialogue as they listen to mood music. Alternatively, the facilitator might present a cartoon, a poster, or a brief sketch to give a different perspective on an issue that concerns the group. In addition, paper, pencils, or crayons might be passed out so that the participants can visually express themselves.

In many ways, wrap-ups are similar to warm-ups. Both are designed to help the participant express and integrate the significant issues and feelings that have emerged through the material and dialogue. And in both cases, the facilitator is responsible for providing appropriate materials and for allowing enough time for the activity to be completed. Results (drawings, responses to the cartoon or poster, etc.) may or may not be shared, depending on timing and other circumstances.

9. Creative writing should be singled out from other wrap-up activities. We will discuss the facilitation of this form of material in detail in the next chapter, but for now note that bibliotherapists draw on what they know of the group to decide what form the original writing should take in a given instance—be it a one-word or a group poem, or an unstructured or structured individually composed piece.

10. Developmental groups in particular might make it a policy to use a form of closure similar to that employed by Otto (1973) in his group-therapy sessions. That is, all participants are asked to verbally identify what in the session seemed personally most valuable: Was there something that added to their self-knowledge or triggered a thought that they wanted to reflect on further?

Otto also suggested that members plan some action they might take in light of their new self-perceptions. Group members may decide to keep a notebook in which they record what they learned at each session as well as the action they planned. In a strongly supportive group, some time at the beginning of each session could be devoted to having members report on their actions.

There is a full repertoire of ways to bring a session to close. But whatever strategy is chosen, the bibliotherapist should work to help participants see that the issues under discussion are not closed—that the process of growth and self-understanding is never finished. When the participants meet again, their understanding should be a little different; in other words, some growth should have taken place.

Overview of Strategic Considerations

Each bibliotherapy session is unique (as is each facilitator); hence, although many appropriate strategic modes of proceeding and types of interventions exist, there is no one correct strategy that fits all cases. Still, we can summarize the main considerations a bibliotherapist must take into account.

- Be aware of what you are comfortable doing so that you can be genuine in your behavior.
- Know your participant or participants.
- Determine what the individual or group members are comfortable doing. Encourage and develop growth within the range of possible responses.
- Be aware of the point at which the member(s) will be able to go beyond the previous pattern of response to more trusting levels.
- Be aware of your own generalized goals. Analyze the value of your specific objectives. Examine the ways in which specific strategies further them.
- Examine the themes and strategies you have chosen over a period of time. Allow them to teach you about yourself. If your approaches or materials are chosen from a limited range, your own limitations may bear looking at. Also evaluate how responsive you are to the therapeutic needs of your participants. If you are consistently avoiding a particular issue, be prepared to get supervisory help to deal with the problem for yourself so that you can aid others.
- Remember that your role is to facilitate self-understanding, not to teach or prescribe. Evaluate how well your interventions encourage participants to do their own work.
- Be aware of how much you want or need to use innovative techniques just to prove your own creativity.
- Be aware of your obligation to set boundaries for the behavior and verbal responses of the participants in a way that is respectful of everyone.

STUDY GUIDE

1. List the major strategies for presenting bibliotherapeutic material chosen by the facilitator. Include a specific example with each possibility, drawing on your own experience, the cases cited throughout this handbook, or outside reading. But also consider the circumstances in which it would not be advantageous to use the particular strategy.

2. Cite the major considerations a bibliotherapist must take into account when deciding whether to have members select material in or outside the group setting.

3. Draw up your own list of possible facilitating interventions; then, using your own experience and/or cases cited in this book or elsewhere, identify the instances in which a given form of intervention both would and would not be strategically advantageous.

4. Discuss the importance of closure; include examples.

PRACTICUM

1. Design five warm-up activities for different groups that you have or hope to work with. Explain why you have chosen each one, in terms of specific objectives and probable outcomes.

2. Design five presentations in which complementary materials or realia are used. Specify both the work of literature and the complement used in each case. Then list the objectives you hope to further.

3. Use a videotape of a bibliotherapy experience to take notes on the way the facilitator uses a particular type of intervention (e.g., nondirective questions or remarks, directive statements or questions, silence, etc.) in the course of a session. For each such intervention, (1) evaluate how appropriate it was in the circumstances; (2) evaluate how effective it was; and (3) indicate whether there were any other points in the discussion at which a particular kind of facilitation would have been strategic. In a class situation, each student might choose a particular type of intervention and then share his or her observations.

4. Alternatively, select a segment of tape or video five to ten minutes in length. Note and evaluate all interventions made by the facilitator in that period. Indicate the type of intervention used (directive, nondirective, etc.), its appropriateness to bibliotherapy, and its effectiveness.

FURTHER READINGS

Bandler and Grinder (1975) and Grinder and Bandler (1976) discuss in two volumes their theory of therapeutic communication based on transformational grammar; they also build on some of Bateson's (1979) theories of communication. Although the formal notations at the end of each volume are somewhat technical, the approach itself and the many examples throughout offer a useful approach to interpreting and facilitating dialogue. The techniques are especially valuable for helping participants specify what they mean. Rioch et al. (1976) provide a good textbook for developing facilitating skills. The discussions in Elkins (1979) and Phelps and Dewine (1976) are aimed at improving communication skills and building self-esteem. Both include exercises and techniques that can either be adapted as warm-ups or used in the course of the dialogue. Ballard (1982) also provides exercises that can be adapted for use in bibliotherapy. Meichenbaum and Cameron (1974) study the process of modifying what clients say to themselves.

Pederson et al. (1981) and Hall (1976) present discussions of counseling across cultures that will be helpful to facilitators who must take into account the diverse backgrounds of their participants. Bibliotherapists working with minorities will find Kochman (1981) a valuable analysis of expressive behaviors that are common in Black American culture but that are unfamiliar and subject to misunderstanding by many whites. Gendlin (1971), Forrest (1976), and Maher (1972) discuss schizophrenic patients in terms of language. Related articles in which bibliotherapists describe their experiences with schizophrenics are those by Edgar, Hazley, and Levitt (1969), McKay (1978), and Hallowell (1983). Meissner (1977) provides an awareness of how paranoid individuals process information. Finally, Borriello (1973) suggests techniques to use with patients with acting-out disorders.

10

Facilitating Creative Writing

A developmental group of single parents was presented with the poem "Landscape: February," by Peggy Patrick Miles:

The roadside stands
of summer
are bare—
a snowless winter
failing to hide
the naked boards.
White steps
that held rows
of vegetable boxes
in August
lie blown over now
on the frozen dirt—
paint peeling
without those red tomatoes.

The facilitator read the poem aloud once. After a short silence, she asked the participants to close their eyes as she read the poem again and then to report on the images they visualized as they listened.

As members shared their responses, the warm-up moved naturally into dialogue when several persons reported memories associated with vegetable or fruit stands, regular Sunday outings, and growing tomatoes. One woman talked of her family's ritual of apple-picking every fall. "We did it for years," she said a bit ruefully. "Everyone seemed to love it. But when I suggested it this fall, even my youngest groaned." She was silent for a minute and then added, "It used to be easier to know what to do with the kids—to know what they enjoyed and how and what they were thinking."

The others felt the speaker had hit on an issue they were all dealing with in one way or another. Everyone spontaneously joined in as the dialogue explored the regrets and/or the relief with which they saw changes in family patterns. Several found that the two very different images of the roadside stand made them think of how various matters in their own lives that had once been central seemed to look different now that they no longer were as useful or important.

By the end of the first hour of the 90-minute session, the facilitator felt that the participants needed to reflect directly on what the discussion thus far had meant to each of them personally. So she asked each of the members to write a short poem using a personal image of an experience or object that was significant in the past but whose importance or function had changed.

Everyone, including the facilitator, worked quietly for about fifteen minutes. Then, as little time was left that day, each member simply read aloud his or her poem without comment. The group agreed that the facilitator would photocopy all of the poems, whether finished or not, before the next meeting so that they could discuss each one in turn.

In the end, it took almost two full sessions to get through the poems. Most people talked about why they chose the image they had. One woman had used the time between sessions to write a new version that she felt gave a more accurate sense of what the image represented to her. But most of the others also found that they saw something in their poems they were not aware of while writing. One man said he felt that the short poem form was too compact and wanted to write something longer in prose. Most of the others showed enthusiasm over the prospect of writing further. Several agreed that they would like to try a prose form to voice their feelings about the changes they were going through.

The facilitator suggested that members should start keeping a notebook in which they jotted down feelings or experiences dealing with change. She would not copy these writings, she said, but each member of the group should be prepared to share something from the notebook at a subsequent session. This idea proved so successful that the group regularly spent the first half-hour of their weekly sessions sharing journal writings and then moving to a selected work of literature.

BEFORE OUR DISCUSSION OF PROCEDURES begins, we must look at the implications of using creative writing as a tool for furthering the interactive process of bibliotherapy.

Creative Writing and the Bibliotherapeutic Process

For purposes of convenience, the original writing of participants is often referred to as "poetry." But the terminology must be properly understood. The significance and value of the writing lies in its meaning for the creator, not in its technical merits. The writings are thus to be viewed and accepted, modified or rejected, on the basis of their validity for the writer, rather than on the basis of style or aesthetics.

Accordingly, original writing in interactive bibliotherapy is not only different from poetry as "art"; it is also distinct from the self-directed activity that Harrower (1972) describes in *The Therapy of Poetry* and from the techniques of journal-keeping detailed in Progoff (1975) and Baldwin (1976). All three suggest topics or approaches that might well be used, but the authors do not consider the writing activity as a prelude to a guided discussion. As valuable as such forms of expression can be, we see them as analogous to the therapeutic potential of reading bibliotherapy. In other words, in the interactive mode, the original writings are the material for discussion led by a trained facilitator.

In effect, then, original writing in interactive bibliotherapy tends to have a double catalytic effect. The act of writing in itself involves the steps of recognition, examination, juxtaposition, and self-application. Then, as the written material becomes the material for discussion, the emotions and concepts are processed again.

Logistical responsibilities

The decision to use original writing obligates the bibliotherapist to be sure that writing materials are available. If the meeting room does not have enough table space, clipboards or large books should be provided to support the paper so that the writing can be accomplished in a comfortable way. In most clinical situations, the bibliotherapist will have to arrange to provide such materials. Developmental group members might be asked early on to come prepared at all times with a pen or pencil in case original writing is called for. In that way, the bibliotherapist will need to keep only paper and extra pencils on hand. If a group uses original writing frequently or as the primary source of material, participants can be asked to bring a notebook or folder as well.

The bibliotherapist is also responsible for establishing a good climate for writing. Participants should understand that they will be concentrating on expressing themselves—that no one's effort will be evaluated for handwriting, spelling, punctuation, or neatness. In fact, the facilitator should assure those who are not used to writing that revisions are part of the process. If a word or a line is scratched out and replaced by another, chances are the change represents a new level of meaning or insight, not a mistake.

Comportment also affects the climate. Clinical participants or young children in a group situation may need to be reminded to respect others' needs. In some cases, the group will have to agree on policies about working quietly and on one's own.

Finally, participants seem to write more comfortably when the bibliotherapist personally takes part in the activity. To have one observe while others write exaggerates the difference between facilitator and participant; some persons will see an implicit message that the bibliotherapist considers himself or herself superior to the activity or, worse yet, that he or she is using the opportunity to judge the participants.

At the same time, it is important to recognize the fact that, although anyone able to participate in a bibliotherapy group can benefit from original writing, not everyone will be capable of the physical act of writing. Some participants will be illiterate, others disabled. Still others may have some kind of psychological block. In any such case, the bibliotherapist should not rule out original writing but should arrange to have the participant dictate his or her responses to the facilitator or co-therapist.

When the majority of the group needs assistance with the actual writing process, the bibliotherapist may have to rely on strategies such as group poems, oral recitation, or storytelling. If the equipment is available, tape recorders might be used to transcribe the individual's efforts.

In most cases, however, only one or two participants will need assistance with writing. As illiterate adults are often very sensitive about their disability, the bibliotherapist will have to be careful about the manner in which assistance is offered. Instead of focusing attention on the individual, work out a matter-of-fact statement such as "Some of you may not be comfortable with writing out your work. If anyone would prefer to dictate, I will be glad to write down your poem as you tell it to me."

In any case, when we use the term *creative writing* in this chapter, we mean material generated by the participant, but without specifying whether that material was actually transcribed by the individual or dictated to the facilitator.

Strategies for initiating original writing

There are three main circumstances in which the bibliotherapist uses original writing.

1. Occasionally, the facilitator asks for a written response immediately after the bibliotherapeutic material is read or viewed. In the subsequent dialogue, the primary material is filtered through the written spontaneous response. This technique is advantageous when the facilitator wants to be sure that participants are responding personally rather than being influenced

by others in the group. But the strategy is probably most effective with experienced participants who are already attuned to making a genuine feeling-response.

2. Very often the bibliotherapist will use creative writing as a way for each participant to make a personal statement, state a reaction, or create a synthesis of what he or she got out of the material and the dialogue. The assignment may be as simple as a single phrase or sentence or as elaborate as a poem or brief story. So, too, the responses themselves may be shared and discussed, as they were in the opening vignette. Alternatively, they may remain a private way to bring the session to closure. One advantage of this strategy, in any case, is that the preceding dialogue is almost certain to offer some kind of focus for the writing assignment.

3. Finally, creative writing may be used exclusively as the material for a bibliotherapy session. As we saw in the series of sessions reported in Chapter 5, the facilitator can bring in a variety of materials but periodically devote two or three meetings to discussing the participants' own writings. Or, as in the case of some developmental groups, the facilitator can start with the understanding that *all* the material will be produced by the participants.

In any of the three aforementioned strategies, the bibliotherapist should be prepared to deal with participants who protest that they can't write. Sometimes it will be enough to reinforce (with both verbal and nonverbal messages) the fact that genuineness is the only criterion for evaluating the writings. As mentioned earlier in this chapter, creative writing is a new experience for many. In addition, those who have had negative school experiences may well feel threatened by the prospect of expressing their thoughts on paper. They need to feel confident that in bibliotherapy the purpose and the evaluation of the writing are distinct from classroom assignments. Repeatedly, we have observed individuals who, although they seemed intimidated initially, were able to produce very significant material once they felt assured that their efforts would be evaluated only in terms of genuineness. Moreover, these persons not only gained new insights into themselves, but their success gave them an intense feeling of accomplishment as well.

A strongly supportive climate is the real key to overcoming the resistance that stems from unfamiliarity with the task. One community mental-health center, for example, set up a writing group deliberately composed of individuals who were the poorest communicators in other therapeutic programs at the center. Each session opened with forty-five minutes of writing on a specified theme, and everyone—including the psychiatrist facilitating the group—was expected to work. Then the next forty-five minutes were spent sharing and discussing the writings or verbal reports. Other staff members agreed with the psychiatrist in charge that most of the patients were ultimately better able to communicate as a result of their membership in this group.

When the writing is the primary material of a meeting, the bibliotherapist may sometimes warm up the participants with a focusing activity. Taylor (1980) describes some simple but useful activities of this sort. Other loosening techniques are included in writing manuals, such as that by Rico (1983).

Now and again, a participant may express dissatisfaction with the proposed theme or form of the writing assignment. If the objection seems genuine, the bibliotherapist should allow any reasonable substitutions. However, if the resistance is deep-seated and/or represents an inappropriate attention-getting manipulation, the facilitator will have to evaluate quickly what strategy is most likely to bring about an appropriate response. If the motive seems to be to get attention, the best strategy is to respond quickly and firmly with a comment such as, "Remember our rules are that no one has to write, but we would be glad to hear what you have to say," or "We all will learn more how each of us feels about loneliness if we share writings on the same subject."

If the individual is really unwilling to deal with the theme or form, the bibliotherapist might suggest, "I can see this choice of topic makes you uneasy. Perhaps we can learn something if you try to write out why you do not like the idea of dealing with it."

Other alternatives can be offered as well. If the structure of the material has not been specified, suggest that the participant try a cinquain or anagram—forms that almost write themselves. Maybe the individual would find it easier to start with a sketch or a mental image that could then be described in words: "If you shut your eyes and think 'wall,' what mental image do you get? Now try to write a description of when and how you might encounter that wall." Or, "Draw a picture of a lonely person; then write a story about your drawing."

On the other hand, people who freeze up when faced with a specific assignment need to be told not to put all of their energy into getting the form "right" or into worrying about whether or not their approach "correctly" reflects the topic. The most important thing is that the product be genuine. Moreover, as useful as it is to help participants express themselves, the facilitator should not cajole or force participation.

The bibliotherapist may have a very different problem in some developmental groups whose members are highly literate. Those who write a great deal or are very anxious about achieving may find it difficult to express personal feelings. Thus one person may become so concerned with conforming to the structure that he pays little attention to the content; someone else might feel frustrated because her poem didn't meet her aesthetic standards. It may help if the facilitator cuts down the time available to do the writing or deliberately uses an unfamiliar or less structured form to loosen up such people. But, again, the facilitator may have to ask the participants to discuss the function of the writing process in bibliotherapy and to look at the way some people may be using their facility with words to avoid personal feelings.

Facilitating discussion of creative writing

When creative writing is the material for bibliotherapeutic dialogue—either alone or in conjunction with other material—bibliotherapists should use the same interventions and strategies for examining the work as those described in the previous chapter. However, we should note in particular several approaches that are especially productive for dialogue about self-generated material. First, many persons will find it useful to reflect on how they felt *as they wrote* or to explore what led them to choose the particular image or attitude used in the finished piece. Second, given the possible time lag of one or two sessions before an individual's contribution is discussed, the facilitator can take advantage of the fact that something new often happens between the writer and the writing when the original writing is allowed to ferment before the dialogue. When an individual says, "I'm not sure now what I had in mind when I wrote this," or "This does not really say what I meant," a dialogue in which this discrepancy is explored can lead to significant self-understanding.

We indicated before that the facilitator normally joins in the writing activity. This participation should be genuine. Indeed, the created product often has real personal significance for the facilitator. However, it is not always advisable for the bibliotherapist to share his or her work. In general, it is best to do so only if group members indicate interest. In most cases, too, the bibliotherapist would use his or her own writing as material for the others to respond to and thus would have to be careful to maintain objectivity about the way in which others are likely to understand the piece.

Major Forms of Creative Writing

Now that we have examined the procedures for using creative writing as the material for bibliotherapy, we can look at some of the many forms such writing can take. Note, again, that although the examples specify "writing," we assume that the facilitator will take dictation, call for oral recitation, or use some other appropriate strategy with participants who do not write themselves.

Poetry

As we pointed out earlier, we understand the term *poetry* in creative writing to have a rather loose meaning. But even so, we can distinguish a number of distinct forms that a poem might take.

One-word poems. Those who are uneasy with writing or verbal expression often feel more at ease if they begin writing by using only one word. Even that chosen word will have significance, of course—but the main goal of this exercise is to help build a sense of pride.

The facilitator invites participants to write by saying, "Could you write just one word on this piece of paper to tell us what you feel about what we just heard [or saw on film]." The facilitator should be somewhat unobtrusive the first few times this strategy is used: Initially, hand out plain sheets of paper and pencils as matter-of-factly as possible. Then, when the members are used to being asked to write, offer them a choice of colored paper and contrastingly colored pens so that the way in which the word is written becomes part of the expression. The activity can become even more complex if the facilitator asks the participants to do a collage of letters cut from magazine ads and glued to cardboard.

Group poems. The group poem is a good strategy for developing both awareness of others and group cohesiveness. It can be initiated as a first response to the presented material, as a method of closure for the dialogue, or as a way of creating a text to be discussed. The bibliotherapist asks each member to contribute a single word or a line that reflects a response to the material, the dialogue, or a specified theme. Once the contributions have all been made, the facilitator may then ask if the members would like to rearrange their order to suit the group as a whole. In addition to the therapeutic results of selecting an appropriate word or phrase, group poems can build social skills. For example, participants may have to exercise patience and respect for others when one person hesitates over what to say.

When group poems are used in clinical bibliotherapy, the therapist may use a blackboard or flip chart to record different contributions. Retarded and regressed mental patients often have limited powers of retention. Accordingly, it may happen that when the facilitator rereads a group poem written during a previous meeting, participants are surprised (and often pleased) to discover that they themselves produced the material. The group effort thus becomes a productive stimulus for more dialogue.

Rance and Price (1973) describe in detail the techniques they evolved for writing group poems in a psychiatric hospital. But group poems can be used with developmental groups, too. This is an effective technique to use not only with children or persons with limited writing skills but with other groups as well. For example, group efforts are often productive for adults who have difficulty expressing their feeling-responses in writing or who fear individuating themselves to the degree demanded by sharing a whole poem of their own composition.

Structured forms. If participants are anxious about what theme or aspect of a theme they should choose and what form they should use, self-expression can be made easier by a clear structure to follow. Furthermore, the demands of a structure sometimes force writers to consider phrasings that would not otherwise occur to them. At times, the process of weighing one wording against another can reveal significant feelings. By the same token, certain forms are very compressed and thus stimulate the participant to sort out what is most important and meaningful. As we have seen, poetry is the distillation of emotion or experience. An image can capture a feeling that it would be difficult, if not impossible, to put into prose or to speak aloud. Finally, as some of the structures we describe are fairly obscure, individuals who might otherwise consciously try to imitate a master of the form will have no preconceptions about what a "good" cinquain or tanka is.

Yet as advantageous as the structure may be, bibliotherapists are usually fairly general in their descriptions of the forms. They should never reject a work because someone failed to follow the form exactly. However, the facilitator might occasionally suggest that revising a poem can refine the individual's own understanding of the theme. Some facilitators feel strongly that guidance in rewriting is part of the therapy itself.

Creative writing can take any one of a number of forms. For instance, the bibliotherapist might ask participants to give their poems some structure by using a *rhyme scheme*. Usually the facilitator would direct participants to use any rhyme. However, in special cases, the facilitator might suggest using the same scheme as that found in a poem that has served as the primary material for the session. Koch (1973), for example, has used this strategy.

Haiku and tanka. These are two Japanese forms whose essence is at once concentrated and abbreviated: Both suggest much more than they say. In addition, they usually draw on nature imagery or suggest delicate emotions. Technically, a haiku is made up of seventeen syllables in three lines (5, 7, 5). Its brevity makes the form look easy to some, but in fact the compression can make haiku very challenging. The following two examples written in a bibliotherapy group show the variety allowed by the haiku:

a boy, at camp—
alone with mosquitos—
in steamy pup tent.

Fall evening, fall night
the sliced half-moon is tilting
its darkness to light

The tanka, or waka, is somewhat longer in that it consists of thirty-one syllables divided over five lines. N. H. Lawrence (1978), an American who lived in Japan for many years, adapted this form for use in English. Although it does not use a nature image, the following poem by Neal Henry Lawrence is the kind of expression that could be powerful for a bibliotherapy session:

Each standing, pressed tight
In crowded train, one body
Warm against another;
Mask of each one hiding own world,
Alone and oblivious.

Cinquain poetry. This form is related to haiku and tanka but was invented by the American poet Adelaide Crapsey. It, too, depends on brevity and juxtaposition of images. Its five lines can be described as being made of stresses, syllables, or words. Raymond Luber (1976) has successfully used this mode with both hospitalized and outpatient mental patients. This is the format he has adopted:

Content	Length
Line 1: Title—a noun	1 word
Line 2: Describes the title	2 words
Line 3: Action words or phrases about the title	3 words
Line 4: A feeling about the title	4 words
Line 5: Refers to the title	1 word

These examples, produced in a bibliotherapy training workshop, illustrate the form.

Illness
This flu
Coughing, aching, sneezing
Why this betrayal
body

Love
strong bond
Sharing, comforting, listening
As necessary as bread
Feeling

Trotzer (1977) uses a cinquain-like form but adds another element so that the participant first generates *lists* and then chooses one to three words from them. This "poem of the self" calls for five lists of words or phrases (what the person looks like, acts like, likes to do; what nouns remind others of the person; names of places they would like to be. Specifically, the person writes his or her name at the top of the paper, composes five lines by choosing one to three words from each list, and ends with a nickname at the bottom. Gladding (1984) adapted this format by having family members work together: The first line is the family name; the second is composed of the individual members' first names; and the third through eighth lines uses words from the lists that all members have agreed on.

Alphabetical poetry. In this form, a structure is imposed on the first word of each line. The facilitator might direct the participants to work out a poem using initial words that follow in alphabetical order. Anagrams are a common variation of this form in which the first letters of each line spell out a theme word—any word that has meaning for the participant, such as a concept, a person's name, or a location. For example, one participant wrote

C *Coming*
O *Out of that glowing*
M *Moment, I*
F *Forgave each and every*
O *One I had*
R *Refused to tolerate*
T *Till then.*

In another case, Chavis (1984) asked the participants in a developmental group to write out their mothers' names with a phrase or word for each letter; after a discussion, participants were told to put down their own names, again with a word or phrase. The discussion that followed indicated that the members had found the paired writing a rich stimulus for comparison, contrast, and insight into their feelings about themselves and their mothers.

Parallelism

This mode is a simplified form of the internal dialoguing recommended by Progoff (1975); it is based on the kind of deliberate reiteration found in lines from psalms, such as "O God come to my assistance; O Lord, make haste to help me." To initiate writing using this form, the facilitator asks members to think of a phrase that spontaneously occurs to them when a specific word is mentioned. For example, the facilitator might say,

"Choose a color that you like [or one that you don't like]. Write it down."

"Now write a phrase that explains how you feel about the color." Allow the members enough time to respond; then continue:

"Write down something else that came to your mind as you were making the first response."

Again allow time for writing. Then close the activity by saying, "Now, is there anything else you want to write about that color or your feelings about it?"

Allow another moment of productive silence before initiating the discussion. As all members are responding to the same initial word, there is great potential for productive juxtaposition. For instance, members who are very self-absorbed may develop an insight into the way their own reactions are shared with some and quite distinct from others.

In any case, the simplicity of this technique is part of its effectiveness. It would be counterproductive, for example, for the facilitator to offer more than one word at a time, as clarification comes from the repeated confrontation with the same concept. However, the bibliotherapist does make strategic decisions about the kind of word to be used initially. Thus, the first few times the technique is used, the facilitator should limit the key word to concepts that most people respond to simply because these concepts are ordinary and personal but not intimate. For example, almost everyone will be able to write down a favorite time of year, season, bird, flower, type of weather, or book. Then more intimate subjects can be introduced gradually, including words relating to familial relationships, emotions, and interpersonal or work issues.

Parallelism has been a particularly effective way to approach a significant issue that the facilitator feels was touched on but not dealt with adequately in a session. In this case, the facilitator would open the next session by using the parallelism technique with a word related to that issue—perhaps a word used in the literature or dialogue. Depending on the kind of dialogue that results, the entire session may be centered on the parallelism poems generated by the participants. Alternatively, the facilitator may wish to use the writing as a warm-up activity and follow it up with another poem, story, article, or film that delves more deeply into the same concept.

Unstructured writing

Although structure is freeing to some, it is threatening or confining to others. At times, the facilitator may feel that the participants are ripe for the kind of self-analysis writing can bring about but that a structured assignment would distract from the reflective process. Then again, some facilitators will be more comfortable than others in giving directions for structured writing. In other words, there are many reasons for which the bibliotherapist would issue a simple invitation to write.

If the writing is to be the material for the session, the invitation can be phrased like this: "We agreed to write at this meeting. The topic you chose was 'Tears.' Let us each write whatever we wish about the theme. When I notice that most of us are finished, I will announce how much time the others have to finish, and then we can discuss each of our writings."

On occasion, a session may be closed with the proposal that members agree to take some time before the next meeting to write something about the issues in that day's discussion. These writings would then be presented and discussed at the next meeting.

When left free to choose the structure of their writing, participants tend to respond initially in ways that reflect their background. Those who are not used to writing often write very little at first; others turn to rhyming because it is a structure they strongly associate with poetry. Others quite consciously structure a story with a beginning, middle, and end. However, as time goes on, the unstructured writing tends to become more and more a simple expression of feelings or a brief personal thought that approaches free verse.

Storytelling

At the beginning of the chapter we suggested dictation or oral recitation as an alternative form of self-expression for those who have trouble writing. But even when participants are comfortable writing, the facilitator might decide to take advantage of the somewhat different reflective and organizational processes involved in oral presentation.

In some cases, a story can be used as a warm-up; "Today let us begin by having each of us tell a joke that we think is especially funny." Or the proposed story line may build on a particular piece of material: "Let us go around the group and have each of us tell a story of a time when we felt like the boy in the story we just heard."

But storytelling can also be an especially powerful device for generating bibliotherapeutic material. We have already referred to Gardner's (1969, 1971) technique of mutual storytelling. Chambers (1977) discusses both theory and techniques for oral storytelling and for creative dramatics. As with written work, participation by everyone in a given group is likely to take more than one session. Of course, although everyone can be encouraged, no one should be forced to make a contribution. It has been our experience, however, that once they feel confident that the climate is accepting, most people can tell a story of some sort. As is true with any form of creative expression, some persons will be much better able than others to produce a piece that is pleasing to the listeners. But it is the facilitator's responsibility to make it clear that *every* genuine contribution has value precisely because it is a personal expression and a tool for growth.

The "story" can take many forms. In some cases, the facilitator will ask for content that is clearly imaginative but will draw out deeply felt personal feelings or issues: "Take a few minutes to think of an animal fable with a moral that you feel is important. You may want to use one you have read or make up one of your own"; "Tell a story in which you are granted three wishes"; or "Let's have each of us share the fairytale or story that we remember best."

But stories do not have to be fantasy oriented. The noted mythologist, Joseph Campbell, points out that "telling the story" of one's life is integrative and expanding for adults as well as children (1976, 92–93). At the same time, we have found that participants consider it much easier to tell a story than to disclose their feelings in a more abstract way. For example, people who fall back on vague replies to a question such as "What pleases you [or what troubles you]?" respond readily if they are asked to tell a story of a family holiday or other occasion that they have especially enjoyed. We will look in more depth at the value of stories that come out of experience in our discussion of autobiographical expression.

Strategies that specify content

Autobiographical material, journals, and story starters can be used to specify the content for original writing. Although each of these modes could grow out of or be used in conjunction with other texts, autobiographical material in particular tends to provide more than enough material to sustain the dialogue on its own.

Autobiographical sketches. Such life reviews are productive for virtually everyone. Aging individuals, for instance, are often very aware of the interplay between their past and present. But younger persons also need to reflect on their strengths and on coping patterns they have used to deal with previous crises as well as on the feelings they have about the past that affect their present behavior (Butler 1977; Keen and Fox 1973; L. Allen 1981; Meyerowitz and Driskill 1975; Ponzo 1974).

The invitation to write in this mode can be very general: "Everybody has an interest in his or her own background. Sometimes we don't pay enough attention to that. Let us look at our own past. Just write something that comes to your mind and heart." If members seem confused or uncertain by this nondirective approach, the facilitator can offer some kind of starter such as "What is the earliest memory you can recall?" Or, "Do you want to write a letter to someone who was a part of your life?" The letter may be addressed to someone living or dead. Alternatively, the facilitator might suggest that the letter be addressed to the participant himself at a different time—either in the past or in the future. The assignment can be made even more specific for those who still have trouble deciding what to write about: "Write a letter to the self you were ten years ago, giving advice on how to deal with a problem that worried you then."

Autobiographical memories can be taped as well as written down. In fact, because one memory often evokes another, it is sometimes easier to "talk out" memories than to write them down. On the other hand, the writing will sometimes stimulate a useful kind of organization. In this connection, note that bibliotherapy does not call on a different type of memory from that used to produce oral history. However, once the memory has been expressed, the focus is different. In a bibliotherapy group for aged participants, for example, the directed dialogue would explicitly use the memory to build on strengths, to give each elderly person a sense of having led a unique and valuable life, to help point up patterns, and to integrate the past with the present.

Perhaps one of the most discerning analyses of the growth potential that can result from a life review can be found in Helene Deutsch's (1973) description of her own experience in writing her autobiography and the meaning it held for her. Deutsch found that her pleasure in the writing did not come from knowing herself or even from correcting errors or wrongs. It lay in the memory process itself—in the intense emotions that arose as she looked again at those she had loved or hated in the past.

Deutsch's observations offer valuable insights into the way most people's memories emerge. For example, she says that she found it easier to speak of the past than of the present. This is often true for elderly persons, and it may be so for others who are still young. Deutsch also noted that seemingly irrelevant memories intruded into her train of thought, making it impossible to follow a logically controlled path. She knew to expect this in psychoanalysis, but now she felt that virtually any situation in which the usual controls of consciousness are relaxed may produce this lack of formal logic. It follows that bibliotherapists should not interpret loose associative rambling as a sign of senility or as an indication of loss of alertness, nor should they attempt to force what seems to them to be a logical progression on a fundamentally associative process of thought.

As she worked on her autobiography, Deutsch also noticed that harmless, minute incidents sometimes took on lasting significance. Indeed, she occasionally learned more about herself from these small recollections than she had from psychoanalysis: "I have come to the conclusion that memories loaded with guilt feelings offer less resistance if they are called up in the course of autobiography as an objective, historical report on oneself" (Deutsch 1973, 15–16). Finally, as she looked back over her life, Deutsch noted recurrent pattens that knit together her childhood, maturity, and old age. In short, she found that the emotional patterns she observed at the time when she was writing were a continuation of those of her childhood.

The bibliotherapist may thus decide that it would be helpful for an individual to trace such patterns of continuity. But it is not always necessary to do so; as Deutsch testifies, the memory process itself and the intensity of the emotions aroused can generate a significant experience and increase one's self-understanding.

Journals. Another valuable way to examine the self is to keep a journal. This form differs from autobiography in that it does not deal with memories.

Rather, a journal records reflections on and feeling-responses to present, personal experiences.

Before discussing the various ways in which journal-keeping can be initiated, we should point out that both autobiographies and journal entries are much more inherently intimate than other forms of creative writing. As we have said repeatedly, no one should be forced to share such material, although, in most cases, everyone should be encouraged to do so. Clearly the bibliotherapist should plan this activity only for groups that are cohesive and whose members show confidence in and support for one another. Journal-keeping could also be shared in one-on-one bibliotherapy sessions.

We have already noted that some of the structured techniques suggested by Progoff (1975) and Baldwin (1977) can be adapted to bibliotherapy. Fincher (1975) gives a user's perspective on journal-keeping, whereas Jacobs (1970) discusses the use of journals for development of creative thinking in children.

As we saw in the opening vignette, members of a bibliotherapy group can all agree to keep journals, and the selections from those journals can become material for discussion. Yet even when journals are not involved, the bibliotherapist can use techniques such as Progoff's "dialoguing." Progoff suggests that each participant choose a person, a dream, or an event that seems meaningful and then carry on a conversation with this important aspect of one's life to see what can be discovered about one's self. In other words, the technique calls for a sort of internal role-playing, with the self taking both parts. By recording the dialogue in writing (or perhaps on tape), the individual can then look back over his or her own thought processes. But here, too, the bibliotherapist will have to decide whether it is more advantageous in a given case to have the dialoguing done in a group setting or in private. As we indicated, "parallelism" is one possible modification of this form.

Resources

The ideas and techniques we have given here just touch on the many possibilities for stimulating original writing. Facilitators who have been English teachers may have a file of creative-writing assignments that they can adapt to bibliotherapy. Others may consult books on writing for ideas and models. In particular, bibliotherapists may want to start a file of what language arts texts call "story starters." As the term suggests, and in the simplest form, the first line or paragraph of a story is given and members are asked to complete the story. However, there are endless variations that can be productive in bibliotherapy. For example, a problem situation can be outlined and participants would be asked to write a solution. Or, as Bernstein (1981) has described it, pictures cut from magazines can be employed to make up pictorial essays that the participants then use as a stimulus for discussion.

Other bibliotherapists have also picked up on the creative-writing technique of using pictures of some sort to stimulate writing. In some cases, the facilitator will ask everyone to write about the same picture; at other times, the participant will select one photo from a group on a specific theme (i.e., everyone will look for a picture of a face that appeals to them or reminds them of someone, or of a house they would like to say something about, etc.). Alternatively, the selection can be made from a random assortment. In the 1970s, Bantam Books issued a series of paperbacks called *Stop, Look, and Write* that combined pictures and short assignments. For example, Sohn (1969) provides more than seventy-five photos along with suggestions for effective composition assignments. Bibliotherapists will be able to use some of these assignments as is; others need to be adapted to focus more directly on a personal feeling-response rather than on objective description. Facilitators can also build their own files of photos and pictures.

As in other manuals for writing, Sohn stresses the importance of being exact. However, the process by which participants are urged to detail looks, smells, tastes, sounds, and physical feelings is not just a part of effective writing; sensory impressions are a real part of emotional life as well. Very often, as such details are specified, recognitions will be released that can then be examined, juxtaposed, and integrated. Original writing in which the facilitator explicitly encourages development of sensory details can be an excellent tool for this release. In *Mind Play*, for instance, Singer (1976) describes "imaging," which uses oral expression to draw out such details. Bibliotherapists may want to use a similar strategy as material.

Furthermore, in the course of any bibliotherapeutic dialogue, such imaging is sometimes the most effective way to help a participant truly examine a feeling or response. "You seem to be having trouble saying exactly why you were happy that day you went fishing. But tell us more about the day. Was it warm? Do you remember what the sky looked like? Can you describe the fish you caught, or what it felt like to reel it in?"

Kenneth Koch is a poet who has extensive experience teaching writing as a self-emancipating exercise. Although he does not see himself as a "therapist," his techniques are readily adapted to bibliotherapy. In *I Never Told Anybody: Teaching Writing in a Nursing Home* (1977), he describes the techniques he used to get elderly persons involved in writing. Koch's first book, *Wishes, Lies and Dreams: Teaching Children to Write Poetry* (1970), has been invaluable as well—both to many English teachers and to bibliotherapists. Another of his books, *Rose, Where Did You Get That Red?* (1973) is especially helpful in that it recounts the techniques he used to introduce adolescent boys to such classic poets as John Donne. His approach has been adopted successfully for clinical groups.

Stephen Joseph edited a selection of writings by ghetto children in *The Me Nobody Knows: Children's Voices from the Ghetto* (1969). We have found the title alone—"The Me Nobody Knows"—to be worthy of a stimulating assignment. In addition, participants who come from a ghetto background have responded well to rewriting the ideas of one selection or another in their own words, and showing how they agree or disagree with the viewpoint in the original.

J. G. Welch's *Topics for Getting in Touch: A Poetry Therapy Sourcebook* (1982) is a source of many techniques designed to get people involved in writing. Neither Rico (1983) nor Vail (1981) was designed specifically for bibliotherapy, but both are representative of creative-writing sourcebooks whose ideas can be adapted. K. F. Wiebe's *Good Times with Old Times* (1979) also provides suggestions for stimulating memories for purposes of autobiographical writing or taping.

In her introduction, Welch makes a point that applies to any writing technique used bibliotherapeutically: The act of self-expression does not always lead to therapeutic self-understanding as such. Nevertheless, the facilitator can use the dialogue to extend the activity into insight. In other words, in bibliotherapy, creative expression becomes the material for an interactive process.

STUDY GUIDE

1. List the strategic decisions that still must be made once the facilitator has decided to use original writing in a bibliotherapy session. Give examples of one or two conditions that would affect each decision.

2. Report on one of the following studies of life-review, and include a summary of the author's understanding of the use and value of the activity as well as a list of several specific techniques that you consider especially promising: L. Allen (1981), Butler (1977), Deutsch (1973), Kaminsky (1974), Keen and Fox (1973), Meyerowitz and Driskill (1975), Merriam (1980), and Quigley (1981). Members of a class can arrange to share their reports.

3. Using specific examples, summarize the benefits you see in creative writing. Read Lauer (1972) and one of the following descriptions of how creative writing was used by a biblio/poetry therapist: Bell (1982), Edgar (1979), Fogle (1980), Heninger (1977), Luber (1976, 1978), A. Miller (1983), Morrison (1973, 1978), and Waterman et al. (1977).

PRACTICUM

1. Describe a group you are presently working with or hope to work with; then design five strategies for writing with these individuals. Explain what you hope to accomplish in each case.

2. Write an autobiographical sketch of your "Odyssey into Bibliotherapy" and analyze the benefits you derived from doing this.

3. For fifteen minutes write on a theme of your own choosing; use any form you wish, be it prose, a structured poetic form, or free verse. Later, write for another fifteen minutes using a different form. Spend a few minutes analyzing how the difference in form affected your response and the self-understanding you reached.

4. Work in pairs with a fellow student or friend. For about ten minutes, have person A tell person B an imaginary or real story of "My dream of a perfect world." Then have person B spend five minutes describing what he or she heard. Now spend about fifteen minutes discussing the actual listening process—that is, how well B heard and communicated back again. Then reverse the process, with B telling and A responding. This exercise should build both listening skills and awareness of what is involved in oral expression of a story.

FURTHER READINGS

Chevin and Neill (1980) describe a method for rewriting familiar fairy tales as a self-exploratory device. Keen and Fox (1973) discuss the "story" as a way to self-knowledge. Harrower (1972) describes her personal evolution through the "therapy of poetry." Although her approach is quite different from that described in this handbook, she makes many good points about the ways in which writing can clarify self-understanding. Finally, N. Baldwin (1976), Silverstein et al. (1977), and Schecter (1983) describe the various strategies they have used to facilitate original writings in bibliotherapy.

— PART 4 —

THE PARTICIPANT

11

Analyzing the Role of the Participant

A social worker training in bibliotherapy worked with battered women in a shelter. She was using literature as a tool to help the women learn to make the transition from being helpless victims to establishing and defending their identities. The group met twice a week, with some shifts in membership.

In one of the very first sessions, the bibliotherapist had announced that she would be taking some notes during the sessions. Some women looked uneasy, but they accepted the facilitator's explanation that the notes would be used only to help her improve her skills.

Although the women had had little or no experience with discussing literature or examining their feelings, they trusted the staff enough to try any program offered. It took some participants longer than others to speak, but the staff members felt that by using the literature as a tool they could help the women toward a therapeutic expression of feeling about their experiences. When the women simply retold their stories, it took them longer to confront the emotional realities of their pasts.

As the facilitator introduced the material and worked to keep the dialogue therapeutically focused, she noted which members were able to ask for information or to clarify a point they had made. She also became aware of individual patterns of response and assumptions of roles in the dialogue. For example, several of the women were reluctant to speak unless directly addressed. Many interpreted a follow-up question as a criticism and apologized.

The facilitator worked hard to get the members to accept the responsibility for maintaining interactions throughout the group as a whole. She also concentrated on helping the participants learn to focus on their feeling-responses rather than simply on the sequence of events.

The facilitator tried to spend some time after each session to transfer her notes to the various charts she kept for each participant, as she had found that her accuracy was greater when the recording was done immediately. Although she did not always fill out every chart for every person, she tried not to go more than two sessions without making notations on the participants' functioning, responsive patterns, and life-adjustment charts, which she used as the basis for her reports at staffings. She found that the charts brought out patterns of which she had not been conscious but which were confirmed by subsequent observations. Moreover, she found this kind of information critical when planning future meetings.

Thus, although the record-keeping was time consuming, she felt that the insights it provided more than justified the effort.

FROM THE OUTSET, PARTICIPANTS in both clinical and developmental bibliotherapy should understand that they have an active role to play—that bibliotherapy is not something being done *to* or *for* them but, rather, that they themselves are agents of their own growth. Accordingly, each participant shares the responsibility for functioning in the dialogue in ways that contribute to growth.

Task-Supportive Functions

Our discussion of the explanatory and expressive roles that participants take in a productive dialogue is couched in terms of the group. But even in the therapist and single-client setting, the individual participant benefits most from the session if he or she shares responsibility for seeing that real communication takes place. Any time participants do assume such responsibility they can be said to be filling a "task-supportive function." We will list different functions through which participants can further the discussion either by explaining what is meant or by expressing a point of view. However, there is no single model to explain the many possible ways in which these roles can be filled. Rather, the task-supportive roles are assumed at different points by different persons. At times, all the group members seem to share equally the responsibility for keeping the dialogue productive. But it is also possible that one individual in a given group will usually be the one to seek information or that another will regularly articulate connections between different points. In low-functioning groups, participants may be reluctant to assume any of the functions.

In the end, the facilitator is ultimately responsible for seeing that the task-supportive functions are fulfilled. Sometimes it will be necessary to articulate the need for group members to take responsibility for a given role. However, the facilitator should be ready to assume any or all of these functions when necessary.

Explanatory functions

Productive dialogue depends on accurate understanding of both the content of the literature and the discussion of it. We can identify several important functions that serve to facilitate such understandings and the way that participants successfully fulfill them.

Information seeking. In this task-supportive function, the participant becomes able to ask for information whenever he or she is unclear about what the material means or about what another participant is saying.

Information giving. Here, the participant expresses how he or she understands the material and/or relates personal experiences that are pertinent to the dialogue.

Clarifying. Instead of settling for a simple recognition or statement of meaning, the participant raises further questions or probes issues in a way that encourages examination and juxtaposition.

Elaborating. In this function, the participant builds on previous comments by restating them or by giving appropriate personal examples in response both to the bibliotherapeutic material and to what has been said so far in the dialogue.

Expressive functions

Other task-supportive functions have to do with the ways in which issues are presented or put into perspective.

Initiating. In this task-supportive function, the participant becomes willing and able to suggest new ideas or to change the way the material is being viewed so that there are alternate ways to respond in the dialogue.

Coordinating. The participant becomes able to see similarities and differences in the ideas expressed in the course of the dialogue and becomes willing to express these connections when such coordination would be helpful.

Orienting. Although it is neither necessary nor desirable that all participants share the same understanding of the material, the participant should be able to question the direction the discussion is taking when the focus of the dialogue seems to be lost.

Summarizing. The participant can help crystallize the focus of the dialogue by reviewing the various opinions and reactions that have been expressed. The point of such a summary, as we have seen, is not necessarily to agree on a consensus but, rather, to recognize what has been said.

Opinion giving. The participant can share a genuine reaction to the material, including the capacity to express (1) likes and dislikes, (2) agreement or disagreement with the text or with others, and (3) approval, disapproval, or ambivalence.

All the roles we have just listed can contribute to the process of self-understanding in the dialogue about the bibliotherapeutic material. But they do not necessarily have equal importance in any given discussion. In addition, it can be counterproductive for a participant to repeatedly return to just one of the functions. For example, someone who constantly elaborates on a single point could prevent others from exploring the issue in a broader, more significant manner. Thus, although the participants should take up the task-supportive functions in the dialogue as much as possible, the facilitator is responsible for seeing that they do so in a way that is productive.

Nonproductive Roles in the Dialogue

Certain kinds of participation interfere with effective communication. It is important that facilitators quickly and accurately identify these behaviors. Not only should nonproductive interactions be cut off, but participants should also learn to recognize that these behaviors interfere with everyone's ability to grow in self-knowledge.

It can be strategically advantageous to involve others in the group in deciding how to deal with nonproductive functions. As we shall see in the next chapter, participants in a strongly cohesive group may spontaneously perform standard-setting and gatekeeping functions. Whoever the corrective comes from, the bibliotherapist must make sure that everyone understands that controlling behavior does not mean that the emotion that led to the behavior should be denied. Rather, the individual should understand that there are constructive ways to express and ultimately to resolve negative feelings.

Before listing the major forms that nonproductive behaviors take, we should clarify two other points. First, the most extreme forms of these behaviors seldom show up in developmental groups; however, such negative manipulations can take many subtle and sophisticated forms, and both clinical and developmental bibliotherapists should be alert for them. Second, the definitions here are quite summary. We cite examples throughout the text, so we do not reiterate the strategies that the facilitator might use to cope with the behaviors.

Blocking or resistance. There are a number of characteristic ways in which a participant might attempt to block discussion of a painful or uncomfortable issue. Some persons will deliberately pursue a topic or approach that diverts attention from the theme under discussion; others will claim that the issue has no relevance to them or consistently attempt to respond in abstract or strictly intellectual terms. Alternatively, participants may insist that others accept only one way of thinking or refuse to allow certain ideas to be discussed. Many of the other negative behaviors we describe may have their origin in a participant's unwillingness to consider a significant personal issue.

Aggression. Occasionally a clinical participant may show physical aggression, but as a rule, in both clinical and developmental groups, this negative interaction manifests itself through destructive criticism, blaming techniques, belittling, and attacking the motives of others. The hostility often will not be directly connected with what has happened in the group and may be either generalized or directed toward a single person.

Seeking recognition. The participant may try to become the center of attention by dominating the discussion, boasting, presenting extreme ideas, or indulging in loud or excessive behavior.

Dominating. Some participants do not want just attention; they want control. They may try to assert authority by interrupting, correcting, giving directions, or intimidating others.

Special interest. Some participants use every topic or opening to introduce a particular theme, concern, or concept that preoccupies them. Such individuals are usually unwilling to dialogue constructively about their fixations and are equally unconcerned with the fact that their perseverating interferes with others.

Withdrawing. A participant who is unwilling to be in the group or reluctant to face personal issues may use passive as well as active techniques to withdraw from the discussion. For example, some persons will put on a show of indifference, give minimal responses, refuse to participate, or even fall asleep. Others may doodle, read, or carry on obviously private conversations during the dialogue.

Analyzing the Participant's Responses

Goals and observable behaviors

Bibliotherapists find that the documentation of their observations helps them to accurately observe and evaluate the individual participant's growth in relation to the goals of bibliotherapy. The record forms we present later in this chapter point to *behaviors* exhibited by the participant. We have said that it is not possible to evaluate rigorously the way a participant internally achieves the goals of bibliotherapy. Nonetheless, it is possible to chart observable changes in verbal and body language that indicate a shift in self-perception. Note that effectiveness is always measured in terms of personal progress rather than against a standardized norm. For example, in the course of six months in a clinical group, Mrs. Y. went from responding only with brief impersonal remarks to direct questions from the facilitator to spontaneously expressing and discussing her own feeling-responses with other members of the group. She clearly benefited from the experience. But Mr. X. also showed signs of significantly benefiting from bibliotherapy, even though he remained fairly withdrawn. In early meetings, he was not willing even to accept a copy of the material; six months later, he did take the paper, examined the text, and usually gave a fairly coherent response to the facilitator when directly asked.

The record forms presented in the next section provide the trainee with an important guide to the kinds of behaviors to look for in the course of the bibliotherapy session. The first three forms in particular call to mind the kind of unobtrusive measures recommended by Webb et al. (1974). As bibliotherapists become more experienced, they may want to adjust the charts to reflect their own personal styles.

In any case, some form of consistent and uniform record-keeping is essential. At any stage of experience, the discipline of noting specific observations is likely to increase the facilitator's awareness of exactly how the participant responds; at the same time, patterns that might otherwise be missed will emerge. We should also emphasize that few persons either perform or progress in smooth, totally consistent patterns. A participant who is deeply involved in the discussion one week may have little to say at another time. Or someone who was basically positive in his attitudes for several weeks may make nothing but negative remarks for one or two subsequent sessions. In fact, it is precisely because the patterns of behavior do fluctuate that regular and precise records are invaluable.

In addition to sharpening attentiveness, these charts are a critical source of information for the bibliotherapist as he or she selects materials and sets objectives for specific meetings and participants. The charts can also serve as the basis for professional reports and evaluations of the general effectiveness of bibliotherapy.

The facilitator will not find it feasible to do any extensive individualized record-keeping during the actual session, however. All bibliotherapists must develop a personal way of accurately noting developments. Over time, they will tend to sharpen their skills in mentally noting what went on in a session so that they can record their observations immediately afterward. Audio- and/or videotapes make accurate recall and interpretation of a session much easier. These aids are especially valuable both for trainees learning how to write reports and for supervisors doing evaluations.

For short-term groups in which members are present only two or three times, the charts should be kept for every meeting. For long-term groups, notations should be made periodically as changes in behavior occur, as institutional requirements demand, or at least every six weeks. Some bibliotherapists find it convenient to follow a loose rotating schedule so that they can limit record-keeping to just a few members each time.

Standard identifying details are recorded on all of the charts. Note that in correctional institutions, mental hospitals, or treatment centers, the requirements of the Privacy Act make it best to use official identification numbers for participants. In developmental groups, it is prudent to use the participant's initials rather than whole names. The bibliotherapist may also find it helpful to specify the author and title of the material used; in this way, the effectiveness of the selection can be analyzed.

The group functioning record

This form (Figure 11.1) should be used by the bibliotherapist to record how the participant functions in terms of the different productive and nonproductive roles played out during the dialogue. The functions that are listed reflect the definitions presented in this chapter. Bibliotherapists should make their notations as specific as possible. For example, instead of recording "Didn't contribute to the discussion," they should make a note such as "After one remark, sat staring into space, inattentive to the other participants' comments."

The responsive patterns record

This chart offers a systematic way to note and record such points as the frequency of involvement, the intensity of the investment (i.e., the willingness to participate), and, finally, the character of the response in terms of self-understanding.

Two forms of the record follow. The first (Figure 11.2) will be used for developmental participants and for many clinical participants. The second form (Figure 11.3) is intended for use with clinical participants who function at a very minimal level, so that even the way they physically handle the material becomes a significant aspect of the record-keeping.

On the socialization chart, behaviors are ordered from top to bottom, with positive interactions first and negative ones last. It is likely that members of a clinical group will show behaviors toward the lower end of the scale, whereas developmental participants tend to show those designated in the center and upper levels.

The life adjustment record

Although this record (Figure 11.4) analyzes the participant in a broader context, it concentrates on observable behaviors and expressions. Thus it, too, is organized not according to the four main goals listed in our opening discussion but according to (1) how well the individual adjusts to the dialogue in terms of coping skills, reality orientation, and self-esteem; (2) how the participant responds in terms of both self-perception and relationships with

FIGURE 11.1 Profile of productive and nonproductive group functioning

PARTICIPANT________________________ GROUP_______________ THERAPIST______________

Use an "x" to mark the occurrence of the following specific behaviors in the dialogue. Briefly note specifics at the bottom of the page.

EXPLANATORY FUNCTIONS (These further a better understanding of the materials or dialogue.)

	Date Sess	Date Sess	Date Sess	Date Sess	Date Sess	Date Sess	Date Sess	Date Sess	Date Sess
Information seeking									
Information giving									
Clarifying									
Elaborating									

EXPRESSIVE FUNCTIONS (These aid in continuing a coherent dialogue.)

Initiating									
Coordinating									
Orienting									
Summarizing									
Opinion giving									

NONPRODUCTIVE FUNCTIONS (These interfere with dynamic communication.)

Blocking/Resistance									
Aggression									
Seeking recognition									
Dominating									
Special interest									
Withdrawing									

DESCRIPTIONS IDENTIFYING THE SPECIFICS OF NOTED BEHAVIORS

FIGURE 11.2 Responsive patterns in bibliotherapy

PARTICIPANT____________________ GROUP______________ THERAPIST______________

Date	Session	List materials and genre/media used in each session.
	1	
	2	
	3	
	4	
	5	
	6	
	7	
	8	
	9	
	10	

PART I: THE BIBLIOTHERAPY DIALOGUE

For the numbered characteristics in Part I, place an "x" in one space opposite the correct descriptor for each session. The composite will produce a graph of behaviors. A second pattern can also be noted when a "v" or "nv" is placed beside the "x" to indicate whether the observation is based on a verbal or nonverbal reaction.

	Date Sess	Date Sess	Date Sess	Date Sess	Date Sess	Date Sess	Date Sess	Date Sess	Date Sess
1. Frequency of involvement									
Usually									
Sometimes									
Rarely									
Never									
2. Intensity of investment									
Very attentive									
Moderately attentive									
Minimally attentive									
Disinterested									
Shows hostility or resentment									
3. Role assumed in dialogue									
(a) Usually task-supportive									
Usually nonproductive									
(b) Both initiates and responds									
Usually initiates function or responds spontaneously									
Usually responds because of another's initiative									
4. Character of response: toward self-understanding									
Self-affirmative (speaks of good qualities; hopeful)									
Generally affirmative (sees self in good light much of the time)									
Indifferent (does not seem to care about self)									
Negative (speaks often of own faults and failures)									
Nonresponsive (does not join in discussion; little facial expression)									

FIGURE 11.2 (continued)

PARTICIPANT________________________ GROUP________________ THERAPIST_______________

PART II: CREATIVE WRITING (whether dictated or written by the participant)

Place an "x" opposite the appropriate descriptor for each session.

	Date Sess	Date Sess	Date Sess	Date Sess	Date Sess	Date Sess	Date Sess	Date Sess	Date Sess
5. Writing (circle if written between sessions)									
Ré personal strength									
Ré personal problem									
Complete, coherent idea									
One phrase									
One word									
Nonresponsive									
6. Character of writing done (circle if written between sessions)									
Shows personal feeling or insight									
Cognitive response ré context									
Unrelated to context, but showing personal concern									
Very generalized response									
No relation to topic									

PART III: SOCIAL INTERACTIONS

Place an "x" opposite the phrase that most nearly describes the participant's behavior in each session. The composite will produce a graph of behaviors.

	Date Sess	Date Sess	Date Sess	Date Sess	Date Sess	Date Sess	Date Sess	Date Sess	Date Sess
A. Relationship to Others									
Initiates exchanges with other members									
Exchanges freely with other members									
Mentions relationships with others									
Appears aware of others									
Erratically tolerates others									
Never notices others									
Relates with hostile verbals to others									
Engages in disruptive behavior									
B. Relationship to Bibliotherapist (Bib.)									
Relates openly and freely with Bib.									
Initiates open exchange with Bib.									
Usually responds to overtures from Bib.									
Sometimes responds to overtures									
Rarely speaks directly to Bib.									
Avoids eye contact									
Responds with hostility to Bib.									

FIGURE 11.3 Low-functioning participants responsive patterns in bibliotherapy (low-functioning participants are those in clinical settings who need reminders about personal hygiene, have poor time and place orientation, and do not seem aware of others)

PARTICIPANT____________________ GROUP_______________ THERAPIST______________

Date	Session	List materials and genre/media used in each session.
	1	
	2	
	3	
	4	
	5	
	6	
	7	
	8	
	9	
	10	

PART I: GENERAL CHARACTERISTICS OF THE PARTICIPANT

To record observations for Part I, place an "x" in one space opposite the correct descriptor for each session. The composite will produce a graph of behaviors.

	Date Sess	Date Sess	Date Sess	Date Sess	Date Sess	Date Sess	Date Sess	Date Sess	Date Sess
A. Attitudes									
1. In general									
Alert (eye contact, erect)									
Passive (inert body)									
Depressed (negative, sad)									
Erratic (moods up and down)									
Withdrawn (little eye contact, slumps, listless)									
B. In Relation to Self									
2. Personal appearance									
Well-groomed									
Undistinguished									
Unkempt									
C. In Relation to Time									
3. Orientation									
Synchronizes time with society									
Makes no realistic plans for the future									
Lives in the past or unreal present/future									
Confuses past and present									
D. Ability to Concentrate									
4. Attention span									
Consistently aware (eyes alert, body attentive)									
Fairly continuous attention									
Intermittent									
Very short									
Nil									

FIGURE 11.3 (continued)

PARTICIPANT____________________ GROUP_______________ THERAPIST_______________

PART II: RESPONSES TO BIBLIOTHERAPY IN GENERAL

To record observations for Part II, place an "x" in one space opposite the correct descriptor for each session. The composite will produce a graph of behaviors.

	Date Sess	Date Sess	Date Sess	Date Sess	Date Sess	Date Sess	Date Sess	Date Sess	Date Sess
A. Attendance									
1. Manner of attending									
Voluntarily appears									
Encouraged by staff									
Assisted by staff									
Refuses to come									
B. Physical Response									
2. Deportment									
Appears comfortable									
Appears on time									
Tolerates remaining									
Agitated behavior									
Comes and goes									
Leaves									
Leaves in anger									
3. Reaction to material									
Examines with interest									
Keeps and uses									
Looks at									
Erratically relates									
Takes									
Destroys									
C. Dictated Creative Writing									
4. General response									
Dictates complete thought									
Dictates one phrase									
Dictates one word									
Refuses to participate									
5. Character of response									
Shows personal feelings and/or insight									
General response ré context									
Unrelated ré context, but appears to be genuine									
Very general response									
No relation to topic									

FIGURE 11.3 (continued)

PARTICIPANT____________________ **GROUP**________________ **THERAPIST**________________

PART III: SOCIAL INTERACTIONS

Place an "x" opposite the phrase that most nearly describes the participant's behavior in each session. The composite will produce a graph of behaviors.

	Date Sess	Date Sess	Date Sess	Date Sess	Date Sess	Date Sess	Date Sess	Date Sess	Date Sess
A. Relationship to Others									
Initiates exchanges with other members									
Exchanges freely with other members									
Mentions relationships with others									
Appears aware of others									
Erratically tolerates others									
Never notices others									
Relates with hostile verbals to others									
Engages in disruptive behavior									

B. Relationship to Bibliotherapist (Bib.)									
Relates openly and freely with Bib.									
Initiates open exchange with Bib.									
Usually responds to overtures from Bib.									
Sometimes responds to overtures									
Rarely speaks directly to Bib.									
Avoids eye contact									
Responds with hostility to Bib.									

FIGURE 11.4 Life-adjustment record

PARTICIPANT_______________ GROUP____________ THERAPIST__________

Date	Session	List materials and genre/media used in each session
	1	
	2	
	3	
	4	
	5	
	6	
	7	
	8	
	9	
	10	

PART I: OBSERVATIONS ABOUT ADJUSTMENTS

To record observations for Part I, place an "x" in one space opposite the correct descriptor for each session. The composite will produce a graph of behaviors.

	Date Sess	Date Sess	Date Sess	Date Sess	Date Sess	Date Sess	Date Sess	Date Sess	Date Sess
A. Adjustments in Sessions									
1. Coping skills									
Performs very well									
Performs adequately									
Erratic behavior									
Poor adjustment									
Seemingly incapable									
2. Reality orientation									
Performs very well									
Performs adequately									
Erratic behavior									
Poor adjustment									
Seemingly incapable									
3. Self esteem									
Self-affirming									
Positive									
Fluctuating opinion									
Negative self-image									
Seemingly unaware									

B. Further notations: ____________________

FIGURE 11.4 (continued)

PARTICIPANT________________________ GROUP________________ THERAPIST______________

PART II: PARTICIPANT'S RESPONSES IN SESSIONS

To record observations for Part II, place an "x" in one space opposite the correct descriptor for each session. The composite will produce a graph of behaviors.

	Date Sess	Date Sess	Date Sess	Date Sess	Date Sess	Date Sess	Date Sess	Date Sess	Date Sess
A. <u>Self-Evaluation in Sessions</u>									
Capable of accurate self-evaluation									
Optimistic about abilities									
Feels generally OK									
Rarely alludes to self									
Confused about self									
Regards self negatively									
Makes no self-observations									

B. <u>Interpersonal Evaluations</u>
Outside group: ré family or valued others (as reported in group by participant)

Positive									
Adequate									
Negative									
Nothing reported									

For item B, add an "sp" to record a remark made spontaneously.

PART III: FACILITATOR'S EVALUATION OF PARTICIPANT

To record observations for Part III, place an "x" in one space opposite the correct descriptor for each session. The composite will produce a graph of behaviors.

A. <u>Considerations</u>
For continuation of bibliotherapy:

Needs to continue to build self-esteem									
Needs continued stress on reality orientation									
Needs interactions to develop coping skills									

B. <u>Decisions</u> (mark at termination)
<u>Termination of membership:</u>

Has achieved ability to self-evaluate competently									
Ready to benefit from interaction outside sessions									
Is not stimulated by dialogue									
Other reasons (list on separate sheet)									

others; and (3) how the facilitator evaluates the participant's needs and progress.

Coping skills. A person with adequate coping skills can manage everyday affairs with some degree of success. In clinical groups, participants show coping skills by their ability to take care of their appearance and personal hygiene; to get to meals, work, and therapy sessions on time; to enjoy leisure time; and to communicate on a basic level. Developmental group members usually have a wider spectrum of interpersonal, work, and recreational matters to cope with and appear to do so adequately.

Reality orientation. Persons with adequate reality orientation see and understand the everyday world and personal relationships in a way that society would accept as valid and reasonable. Members of clinical groups—especially those who suffer from delusions or paranoia—may have difficulty maintaining reality orientation, whereas members of developmental groups rarely exhibit this difficulty.

Self-esteem. This quality has to do with the way in which a person values him- or herself. The bibliotherapist evaluates self-esteem not only in terms of the participant's verbal expressions but also by looking at personal behavior, interpersonal relationships, and general social competencies. Low self-esteem can be identified by a lack of pride in personal appearance, dissatisfaction with performance, and negative nonverbals such as mumbling, lack of eye-contact, or tics. Low self-esteem is often accompanied by an unrealistically negative estimate of the person's own capacities or achievements. At the other end of the scale, unrealistic self-satisfaction is often manifested by a lack of concern for others.

Analyzing personal strengths

The records we have described are meant to help the bibliotherapist analyze how the various observable behaviors fit into a personal pattern of strengths and divergencies. To aid such analysis, we have drawn up a list of balanced strengths (Table 11.1), which has been designed to help the bibliotherapist decide on materials, interventions, and strategies that will build on strengths and foster personal growth for the participants. This was not an easy list to formulate, however. There is a tremendous variety in what, historically, have been considered strengths (or "virtues"). Classical and early philosophical treatises, for instance, defined prudence and justice as the mental processes by which one gauges action, whereas fortitude and temperance indicated an ability to curb the passions through reason.

More recently, Erikson defined virtues as "certain human qualities of strength . . . by which ego strength may be developed from stage to stage and imparted from generation to generation" (1964, 113). Erikson's list of virtues includes Hope, Will, Purpose, Competence, Fidelity, Love, Care, and Wisdom.

TABLE 11.1 Personality Strengths and Divergencies

Applicable Area	Strengths/ Attributes	Divergencies/ Attributes
Selfhood and self-image	Autonomy/ self-regulated, free, independent	Domineering/ imposing one's will on others
		Role-confused/ lack of clarity about life's responsibilities
	Self-esteem/ objective sense of self-worth	Conceited/ exaggerated opinion of one's worth
		Self-depreciative/ little respect for self
Interpersonal relationships	Collaboration/ working with others; mutuality	Possessive/ jealously opposed to sharing family, friends, or property
		Dependence/ needing others for help or support
	Hope/ believing that which is desired is possible	Pollyannaish/ unrealistically optimistic
		Discouraged/ temporarily disheartened
Self and the world	Competence/ having sufficient skill or capacity to perform adequately	Perfectionistic/ demanding the highest degree of proficiency
		Inefficient/ unable to perform skillfully
	Courage/ ability to face the difficult or dangerous	Rash/ acting without deliberation
		Fearful/ full of apprehension
Self, others, and the world	Appreciation/ ability to intelligently value and enjoy	Biased/ exhibiting unexamined opinions or prejudice
		Callous/ insensitive or hardened
	Humorous/ ability to see absurdity or incongruity in people or situations	Mocking/ using jokes defensively or to embarrass others
		Ill-tempered/ irritable, quarrelsome disposition

In a similar vein, Abraham Maslow (1970, 1971a, 1971b) developed the concept of the "self-actualized" person, whose qualities include a well-balanced sense of humor, a sense of wonder (appreciation), and an acceptance of self (self-esteem) as well as an acceptance of others. Shostrom (1980) also developed a personal orientation inventory scale that seeks to measure self-actualization, whereas Parloff (1969) recommended that outcome measures be devised to gauge joy, ecstasy, peak experiences.

Herbert Otto has been working since the 1960s to develop ways for individuals to look for their strengths and make better use of them. In 1966 he did a study indicating that both adolescents and adults cite only a few strengths when asked to assess themselves, but list a page or more of "weaknesses" or "problems." The Otto Inventory of Personal Resources (1963, 1973) is designed to be kept and used by the individual to make better use of personal strengths.

Human-potential and wellness movements continue to emphasize the development of strengths. Currently, the professional tool entitled *The Diagnostic and Statistical Manual of Mental Disorders III* (DSM III, 1980) provides for some generalized estimation of strengths. In AXIS V of DSM III, estimates are made of the patient's "Highest Level of Adaptive Functioning." However, this section is underdeveloped and unspecified, and it continues to place a primary emphasis on disorder.

J. M. Strayhorn's "A Diagnostic Axis Relevant to Psychotherapy and Preventative Mental Health" (1983) appears to be much more carefully thought out and useful. Strayhorn provides a list of fifty-nine strengths broken down into nine major categories: Closeness/Trusting, Relationship Building; Handling Separation and Independence; Handling Joint Decisions and Interpersonal Conflict; Dealing with Frustration and Unfavorable Events; Celebrating Good Things, Feeling Pleasure; Working for Delayed Gratification; Relaxing/Playing; Decision Making, Organizing; and Adaptive Sense of Direction and Purpose. Although he does not identify himself as a bibliotherapist, Strayhorn does use stories to teach some of these skills to children.

We have drawn on all of these sources to formulate our list of eight areas of personal strength (see Table 11.1)—strengths that are fundamental to a *balanced* personality. Note that emphasis: Our understanding of good mental health works from the assumption that a strength reflects the capacity to function effectively in a way that does not show extremes. For example, a person with the proper level of self-esteem has neither an exaggerated sense of self-worth nor too little respect for self.

Several features of the list should be noted. First, the list shows each strength as a factor of balance. Thus, each of the eight qualities is listed with a brief definition, followed by two characteristics that represent polarized divergencies from this balance. Note that the divergencies can be considered "normal" as well; that is, in themselves these qualities do not necessarily indicate emotional illness given that everyone shows some divergence from the "norm" on occasion.

Second, the choice of terminology pertaining to these traits reflects several evaluations and revisions. In truth, there can be no perfectly satisfactory list. On the one hand, the traits tend to cluster and overlap, such that the chosen terminology indicates one of several possible emphases. On the other hand, those in the helping professions will often understand one term or another in a specialized way. At the same time, some terms were somewhat problematic. For example, Allport (1950), Sorokin (1950), Fromm (1956), and Erikson (1964) are among those who have spoken eloquently of the need for and value of love. However, the term love has such a broad range of connotations that we found it too difficult to establish a single definition or to pinpoint two of the many possible divergencies. Although we hope that our brief definitions will help clarify our understanding of the traits, others may wish to evolve their own list.

The bibliotherapist might also consider using the list of strengths in a direct verbal advisory session with individual participants in a group. In such a session, however, the relationship and the interaction would be quite different from the usual bibliotherapeutic encounter; thus, the facilitator will have to decide whether the session would be appropriate and/or helpful in a particular circumstance. The list in Table 11.1 might offer a format for periodically assessing progress in a one-on-one setting or in a long-term group. Alternatively, the facilitator may decide to evaluate a participant in terms of relevant items on the list as part of the termination procedure for bibliotherapy groups that meet in the context of schools, counseling groups, or other settings in which the number of sessions is fixed. However, participants in developmental groups might have reservations about formal counseling. Then, too, a sponsoring institution such as a public library may not wish to get involved in any procedure that seems to formally characterize patrons, even in this positive way.

Conclusion

The record forms and list presented in this chapter are meant to enhance the possibility of noting increases or decreases in self-esteem and self-understanding and to help in planning future therapy. In addition, they should be used to measure the effectiveness of chosen material and as a convenient system of sharing information with other mental-health workers.

The record forms are the result of trial and error; they represent compromises between the need to devise forms that were concise and reasonably easy to use and the necessity of leaving room for sufficient information. It is our belief that these forms will help trainees in particular to look for and note significant behaviors. However, we do not consider the formulations we have presented to be definitive; as earlier indicated, an experienced bibliotherapist will probably want to adapt the format to reflect his or her personal style. Nonetheless, it is important that you develop some kind of systematized record-keeping that will add to your understanding of bibliotherapy's effectiveness. We invite readers to share suggestions and modifications with us by writing to us in care of our publisher.

STUDY GUIDE

1. Summarize your understanding of task-supportive functions in a discussion situation, and consider the differences between having a participant assume the function and having the facilitator do so.
2. Give three examples of nonfunctional roles in a discussion situation. Suggest possible strategies for dealing with the situation.
3. Summarize the purpose and value of the responsive patterns record.
4. Summarize the purpose and value of the life adjustment record.
5. Read at least one of the discussions of the strengths cited in the text. Draw on the reading, the material in the handbook, and your own understanding of the goals of bibliotherapy to make up a list of strengths you feel can be used to gauge a participant's response to bibliotherapy. Be prepared to explain your choices.

PRACTICUM

1. Use a videotape or recording of a bibliotherapy session to fill out the record forms in this chapter for one participant. Review your notations with your supervisor and/or other students.
2. After you have had some experience working with a group, use the participant's responsive patterns record and the life adjustment record to explore and analyze your own personal feelings toward the participants' attendance, physical responses, socialization patterns, orientation to time, attention span, attitude toward interventions, and so on. Recognize the importance of acknowledging and dealing with the fact that you may find some behaviors upsetting.
3. If you are taking part in a developmental bibliotherapy experience in conjunction with your classwork, use the three record forms as a guide for taking notes after each session on your own responses and on the attitudes and strengths that you see yourself demonstrating. Use these notes to summarize the patterns you see in your own responses.

FURTHER READINGS

The works by Otto (1979) and Hastings et al. (1980) are presentations of the "wellness" movement, which emphasizes strengths and health. As bibliotherapy shares the same emphasis, practitioners may be able to apply the insights in these books. Berchter and Maple (1977) use a personalized workbook approach to help facilitators recognize and better understand the task-supporting functions we have mentioned. D'Augelli et al. (1980) offer a teacher handbook to be used with a workbook by Danish et al. (1980); together they provide excellent exercises for developing skills in observing participants' responses. Finally, Rosenberg (1979) offers a self-esteem scale that has been used with children and could prove a valuable tool in observing changes in self-esteem with low-functioning patients as well as with children in bibliotherapy.

12

Dynamics of the Group in Bibliotherapy

A bibliotherapist was working with a group whose members had chosen to take part in a long-term residential drug unit rather than serve time in prison. These participants had had several months of bibliotherapeutic experience. From initial hostility and suspicion of the facilitator and of reading, the members had grown to trust the bibliotherapist's empathic, nonjudgmental attitude and had come to see that something of personal value could be found in the literature and dialogue. The intensive program had also built a bond among the members, and they trusted each other not to laugh or to mock, but to accept any kind of genuine response.

As the material for one session, the bibliotherapist extracted a passage from T. S. Eliot's Four Quartets *(the last fifteen lines of "East Coker, III"). She did not mention the rest of the poem or try to explain who Eliot was. She also felt there was no need for explaining what a paradox was—the members saw the apparent contradictions as they listened to the poet say that the pathway to finding oneself has "no ecstasy." It is a way of ignorance and dispossession, of knowing only what one does not know and owning what one does not own; the way is one in which "where you are is where you are not."*

After the poem was read, there were a few moments of working silence. Several murmured "Heavy" or "Wow!" but the members lost no time in trying to "cut up the idea," as they phrased it. The young woman who responded first was deeply involved, almost talking to herself. She kept her eyes down, working directly from the lines of the poem to her own experience. "We do have to go through changes; I have a fear of the unknown; I really don't know—ignorance, no ecstasy—it's painful." Looking up, she said to the group at large, "This is really deep."

Several others responded, as much to what they saw in the poem as to the first speaker. At first there had not been too much interaction.

But one young man who frequently asked others to help him clarify points said, "I don't get this line about dispossession. Do you think that means you can't own anything? Like, how about clothes—that's when I knew I was really down—when I didn't care about looking sharp any more."

His question sparked a lively interchange about the importance of material possessions such as cars and clothes. But when two members related the line to the problem of "owning" themselves, the focus of the discussion shifted. Both agreed that you could own yourself only when you had control over your actions. One of the women said she knew she didn't own herself yet because she was too responsive to her environment. A man saw the issue in different terms. He felt that he owned his own feelings and wisdom, then added, after a pause, "With wisdom, if you give it away, share it, you own it better than you did before sharing." At that point a young woman who had not spoken previously was suddenly vehement about the need to dispossess the past: "I do own me, I do control myself. No one can take me away from me. But I can't own anyone else."

Her vehemence led to another working silence. The issue she raised was a significant one for people in a dependency program. Judging by nonverbal behaviors, some members were rejecting her point of view, others agreeing with it.

Time had run out; the facilitator's closing remarks let the statement stand as a personal declaration that invited further examination: "You have expressed something we all need to look at. Next week there will be time to write a response to the poem we have just discussed." In writing up the session, the bibliotherapist felt that even though she had intervened several times to keep the discussion focused, the participants themselves had done much to make this dialogue effective.

IN THE OPENING PARAGRAPHS of this book, we spoke of how the bibliotherapeutic material is like a stranger who makes it possible for the participant to find the treasure of self-understanding. We said that the facilitator can be seen as an "other" who aids in the search, but we noted as well that there can be still others who also contribute to the process of growth. Those "others"—fellow participants in a bibliotherapy group—are the subject of this chapter.

Bibliotherapy as a Group Process

The strengths that are reinforced or developed through group functions are no different from those that the bibliotherapist tries to facilitate. In all cases, the process works through the dialogue about the material. Many points in this chapter have been touched on elsewhere. However, the focus here will be on the ways in which group dynamics contribute to growth.

We have indicated that on practical grounds alone it is more likely that bibliotherapy will be done in a group than in a one-on-one relationship. Moreover, there are definite therapeutic advantages to the way a group functions. At times, the group setting can release a therapeutic experience or insight that might never emerge in a one-on-one interchange. Thus, a clinical participant may be more open to responding to another member who is perceived as a peer than to the facilitator who has been cast as an authority figure. Or a developmental participant will feel freed to acknowledge her feelings because she senses that other members in the group share them.

At the same time, the group mirrors the inherently social nature of the human condition. The process of becoming a fully developed individual inevitably depends on some ability to function effectively in relationships with others. Indeed, as Maslow (1970) has noted: "One necessary aspect of becoming a better person is *via* helping other people." When group members offer support and reassurance or share insights with another, they affirm themselves by reaching out to another.

But before reviewing the therapeutic potential of group interactions, we should note three points. First, what we say here is necessarily summary. Bibliotherapists working with groups must plan to take academic classes in group theory and dynamics. Second, our discussion of group dynamics does not endorse any particular theory about the way functions should be distributed between the leader and the members. Nor do we feel that bibliotherapy should have only supportive-inspirational goals—that is, to the exclusion of psychoanalytical goals. On the contrary, bibliotherapy, to use Lerner's phrase again, is "a tool, not a school," and, as such, it lends itself to different styles of leadership.

In other words, the review that follows *describes* some of the group dynamics without attempting to *prescribe* a particular model of facilitation that will produce the effect or to *interpret* the motives that might lead a participant to assume a function in the dialogue.

Our third point has come up several times. In bibliotherapy, as in other creative therapies, growth is affected by the use of the intervening tool as well by the group dynamics (Armstrong 1979; Zwerling 1979). Thus, in the following discussion, we will pay special attention to how the bibliotherapeutic tool contributes to beneficial group interactions.

The group climate

The facilitator works hard to maintain an atmosphere that is characterized by cohesiveness and acceptance. In such a climate, members recognize that they are gathered together for a common purpose and are willing to support each other in meeting their goals; at the same time, each individual should be able to feel some assurance that any genuine expression of thoughts or feelings will be accepted by the other participants as well as by the facilitator.

As we have seen, the facilitator may have to devote a great deal of effort to build cohesion in clinical groups. But note that this kind of facilitation is not the groundwork on which the goals of bibliotherapy will be met; rather, the goals are met through *interactions* that increase cohesiveness and help communicate acceptance.

For example, the facilitator of a clinical group who involves the participants in accounting for absent members reinforces at least a rudimentary awareness of the third major goal—enlightening interpersonal awareness. The facilitator might ask, "Does anyone know why so-and-so is absent today? We would like to know because everyone is important to us." As clinical participants respond to such remarks over time, they are guided to a real awareness of other members as persons who have identities and engage in other activities. As the group becomes more cohesive, both clinical and developmental participants deepen the level of awareness.

In the same way, we have already seen that some group members are more able than others to carry on a productive dialogue. But as they exercise and improve good discussion skills, developmental as well as clinical participants grow in their awareness of the ways in which they personally relate to others as well as in their understanding that cooperation is necessary for social interaction. In fact, the process has a spiralling effect: The more the group shares the group-building functions of *standard setting, gatekeeping* (seeing that all members are given opportunities to express themselves), and *relieving tension,* the stronger the climate of cohesiveness and acceptance becomes. And as members take initiative in the functions that are even more other-directed, such as *encouraging* (not just tolerating, but responding to others) or *showing empathy* toward each other, both the individual who acts and the person who is helped grow even more aware of the important role that interpersonal relationships play in the way we see ourselves and the way we relate to others.

The benefits we have just noted are characteristic of groups in general. However, the bibliotherapeutic material in itself also contributes significantly to group dynamics. In the first place, the material provides a focus for communication. As we have seen, on a very elementary level the material acts as a common ground. For group members who do not know each other, who share only a limited bond and/or have little internal motivation for developing interpersonal awareness, the material provides something to talk about.

Moreover, the neutrality of the material has several important ramifications. In bibliotherapy the focus of the discussion can be personal without having to become immediately intimate. Members can talk about their reactions to the work itself even when they are not ready to share significant personal issues. At the same time, members can use the material and their responses to it to practice communication skills directly rather than just to identify areas that need work. For example, we have spoken of the difficulty many people have in being precise about their thoughts and feelings. When a bibliotherapy participant fails to voice an opinion about the material in a clear, coherent way, other group members often question or comment. As the original speaker responds and clarifies her meaning, she is getting practical experience and guidance in how to phrase things in a way that others can understand. In other words, the participant does not merely learn to recognize cognitively that "I have trouble expressing strong feelings"; she learns to increase her expressive skills as well.

The neutrality of the material can increase receptivity to selections that specifically direct the attention of the group to issues concerned with cohesiveness. For example, in I. Cutler's "Alone," the speaker identifies with mortar, which feels ambivalent at best about the two bricks it is squashed between. The poem is short, wry, and quite pointed—but it does not aggressively accuse anyone. It is thus less threatening than the direct confrontation implicit in a facilitating remark such as "The resentment some of you seem to be showing toward other members of the group is interfering with the way we are sharing with each other. Let's talk about this."

At the same time, as the bibliotherapeutic material is impersonal, the response to the issue is less likely to be complicated by personal resentment toward either the facilitator or a fellow member who raises discussion of a sensitive point. For example, an individual who has trouble being honest with other people might be able to discuss the Wilkinson poem "Why Do They?" In addition, as we saw in the dramatic case of Lois in Chapter 2, the material often provides enough distancing to free the individual to see how the point of the work applies to self. On the other hand, the same individual might become defensive and withdrawn in response to a direct comment such as "Mrs. Black, you said you think people should be free to make up their own minds, but I notice you refuse to comment further if someone disagrees with you."

Finally, the material provides a common basis for understanding what caused another's reaction, even when the reactions themselves are not similar.

Self-understanding through group dialogue

We have noted the strengths that come from developing a good therapeutic climate, but there are other ways in which the group setting furthers the goals of bibliotherapy. A fair number of examples in this handbook have illustrated how one member's capacity to respond was enriched because someone else shared a response that either triggered or reinforced an insight. Each person brings his or her own themes and experience to the dialogue. Thus a good group discussion releases a much broader range of responses to a single work than any single individual is likely to make. Moreover, as we have seen, the increased capacity to respond often reinforces a movement toward the other goals of bibliotherapy.

Let us briefly review three very significant kinds of insights that members can experience as a result of the varied responses that come from group discussion. First, the dialogue may offer an important insight into the *universality of feelings*; second, a participant may gain a *fresh insight* as he or she realizes that it is possible to understand one topic, image, or issue in very different ways; and finally, the dialogue can provide an opportunity for *reality testing*.

We have already mentioned the first two points a number of times. Regarding the third, there are several ways in which group dynamics can specifically strengthen a participant's orientation to reality. If nothing else, one is more likely to reevaluate an opinion or perception when a whole group of peers questions its validity than when only one person does so. The peer response is particularly significant for a participant who is at a stage of resenting the facilitator's efforts to encourage that individual to be more probing and reflective.

Group dialogue also provides the participant with a forum for getting feedback on possible solutions to a problem or for getting advice about workable strategies that someone else has used to deal with a similar issue. At the same time, as the participants continue to participate in productive dialogues, they tend to become increasingly comfortable with the fact that they do not need to fear or resent differences of opinion. On the contrary, in a climate of mutual respect, important insights come from the process of disagreeing, refining implications, pointing out inconsistencies, and subsequently changing or reaffirming one's position.

In addition to offering a way to evaluate responses to an issue or situation, the group can help an individual grow in self-knowledge and orientation to reality by increasing awareness of the way he or she is seen by others. For example, a clinical group was discussing Hilda Conkling's poem "Butterfly." The poem describes the act of seeing a pink and purple butterfly light on a flower and hearing it say, "Follow"; but the speaker responds "I have to go the opposite way." In this instance, the discussion soon turned to an examination of personal patterns of dependence and independence. One participant was surprised to hear that the others thought him very independent of others' opinions; he saw himself as being obviously hesitant to stand alone. Another participant thought she wanted to be told what to do, but other group members pointed out that she always rejected others' advice. Two people who felt that they were followers did not like that aspect of themselves and wanted to become more independent. They asked the more aggressive members how to develop self-assurance. Their request opened up a general exchange of perceptions about leadership and dependency. In subsequent meetings, the dialogue revealed that some group members integrated what they had discovered from this discussion more effectively than others. But it was also clear that all the participants had learned something about their own realities from the discussion. Indeed, although the facilitator had helped to keep the dialogue focused, the important learning came from what the members shared with each other.

The group setting also permits bibliotherapy participants to increase their orientation to reality by providing *models.* That is, one participant may see another member's reaction as a direct model—in either positive or negative terms: "The problem Mr. Adams dealt with is very similar to what I am going through. I should be able to try the approach he used successfully to resolve it." Or, "When I think about how I reacted when Miss Cann interrupted me, I can see why others might wish that I would wait more patiently for my turn to talk."

We saw a different kind of modeling in the discussion of "Butterfly," when participants directly asked others for advice on how to acquire a certain quality. In other cases, a participant will not be quite so direct but, instead, will observe the way in which the facilitator and/or other group members assume task-supportive functions or express themselves. Eventually, the person will become comfortable enough to try out the behavior.

Finally, members learn about themselves through conscious examination of their interpersonal relationships in groups. For example, Yalom (1975) is among those who conjecture that all group members bring to the group behavior patterns developed in their family structure. The bibliotherapy group offers a relatively safe context in which members can learn to recognize and, if necessary, to modify previous patterns of behavior toward parents, authority figures, or siblings as well as to cope with the emotions of jealousy, resentment, fear, or anger that grew out of those patterns. When the material also directly addresses the issue, the participant has a double chance to work at improving the relationship or the emotion.

Bibliotherapy participants often attest that talking about a work of literature with other members of the group has led them to greater self-understanding. Both clinical and developmental participants have made such remarks as: "Because of the poetry discussion, I've said things in this group that I didn't know I thought and found that they were true"; "I needed to be able to talk about this issue, but I have been unwilling to face it. I am grateful someone else brought it up so that I could begin to come to terms with it"; or, "We have shared so much in our creative writing, we really know each other. I no longer feel alone."

In such bibliotherapy group sessions, the facilitators have often noted that a participant who makes some change as a result of the dialogue will make other changes both inside and outside the group. Something in the group process seems to have freed the individual to take better advantage of other situations and relationships in his or her life.

In short, group dialogue about the literature helps the participants clarify their feelings at the same time that it provides a concrete experience through which they can note and evaluate their personal ways of interacting—of responding to others and of being responded to. That is, in group bibliotherapy the literature and the resulting dialogue are blended with the dynamics of the group to create opportunities for recognition, examination, juxtaposition, and self-application.

Dynamics Characteristic of Stages in a Group

Obviously the precise ways in which the dynamics we have just described work out in any given bibliotherapy session cannot be predicted. Yet one important set of factors can be isolated: Just as there are inevitable stages in any relationship, certain concerns and interactions are characteristic of the beginning, the middle, and the end of any group (Beck 1974). What follows is a brief review of the significant issues and choice of materials for each of these stages.

Early meetings of a group

The actual amount of time it takes any group to develop a sense of cohesion and to settle into a productive pattern depends on factors such as (1) how well the group members know each other to begin with; (2) the kind of bonds or common interests they share; (3) the strength of the members' impetus to use bibliotherapy for growth; and (4) the skill of the facilitator in guiding members to assume and respond to different functions in the dialogue. Thus, a strongly motivated developmental group might settle in after only two or three sessions, whereas it may take up to ten meetings before some clinical groups come to observe such basic procedures as arriving on time or behaving appropriately during the discussion phase.

The first meeting. In all groups, the first meeting is necessarily somewhat *sui generis.* The bibliotherapist will need to introduce him- or herself and the group members to each other. In addition, time must be taken up in reiterating logistical matters such as scheduling (e.g., time, place, frequency of meetings) as well as in summarizing goals and expectations. At this time, the facilitator should review why the members of this particular group have come to try bibliotherapy and whether the membership is open or closed (i.e., whether new members are likely to join during the life-span of the group or whether the membership will be limited to those present). In addition, the facilitator should remind the members that in bibliotherapy the material is a tool for allowing each participant to explore feelings and ideas. Members will be told not to strive for "right" or "wrong" answers but to work at giving genuine responses. In short, although the first session should not be taken up in entirety with procedural matters, members should be given some chance to comment on all of these points before turning to the material for the day.

Significant issues in the early stage. In groups in which members do not know each other, the facilitator should provide opportunities for participants to learn each others' names and identities. In the chapter on strategies we indicated some possible warm-ups. Note, in addition, that the very process of naming oneself or of being named by another—even in the most literal way—can touch on some very significant issues. Thus, when resistance is expressed, the bibliotherapist should not force the matter but, rather, should help others learn the name with a calm remark such as "Very well, John Foster, maybe you can think of a response next time." During the dialogue about the material the facilitator will continue to indicate the personal recognition accorded each person by using the participants' names regularly.

Although naming is not a problem for most people, almost all groups will need to develop some sense of cohesion and mutual trust. The cohesion builds naturally—and quite quickly—when all of the participants are motivated to use bibiotherapy. But some clinical participants are very concerned with issues of dependence and are suspicious of the power of the facilitator or of other group members. Testing behaviors motivated by such anxiety seem to occur most often between the third and ninth sessions. For example, participants will deliberately come late, be absent, or act withdrawn or agitated during this time. As we have seen, the bibliotherapist must use the dialogue to confront and resolve such feelings. In some cases, the facilitator will know of a good selection that lends itself to exploring issues of mistrust and power; at other times, the discussion of boundaries and standard setting will not tie directly into the material but can be brought into the discussion when the issue arises.

In both developmental and clinical groups, it is likely that some participants will be reluctant to disclose their thoughts and feelings, especially in the early sessions. The fear may stem from uncertainty about the trustworthiness of the facilitator and/or the other members in the group. But as the facilitator consistently demonstrates genuine empathy, and as the group climate becomes more supportive, these fears should fade.

However, some persons are deeply suspicious, and others are reluctant to examine themselves honestly. In such cases, the facilitator will select material or direct the dialogue to focus specifically on issues of mistrust or on the value of genuine self-examination.

Choice of materials. Given the issues that are likely to concern new participants, the bibliotherapist should take special care during the first few sessions to select materials that have a broad application but can bring forth personal responses without necessarily demanding deep self-disclosure. At the same time, preference should be given to works that use personal pronouns so that the material itself encourages recognition. In addition, the facilitator should look for items that will have a strong initial appeal and can be readily understood. Finally, as we have seen, the materials should help members address any issues such as trust or cohesion that are important to the group atmosphere.

For example, "The Red Balloon" is a lovely film that many people find both engrossing and appealing in its artistry. For some groups, it will be enough during these early sessions that the members find the bibliotherapeutic material to be simply delightful. But such a film as "The Red Balloon" can also lead to consideration of what freedom means or how persons can cope with isolation, rejection, or persecution.

Bernard Casey's "Look, See" is another poem that initiates the development of sensitivity for life outside of oneself. "Look at the rain," Casey tells the reader—at the tree, at the grass, even at an individual blade of grass, and then go on to look at people, one person at a time. Again, this poem raises very significant issues about respect and concern for others, but discussion could also focus on appreciating the beauties of nature if the group members are not ready to confront the deeper level.

In much the same way, haiku can be very effective in the early meetings of a group. The form is simple but very evocative of mood; moreover, as haiku are usually ambiguous, they seem nondirective. Thus the following example could lead a participant to examine seriously his or her own relationships with others; then again, it might be used as the basis for a more general discussion of attitudes toward group interactions:

A world of dew.
Yet within the dewdrops—
Quarrels.

Sometimes the facilitator will deliberately look for a somewhat light treatment to open up the issues of self-identity, trust, and dependence. For example, a group might discuss Emily Dickinson's "I'm Nobody, Who Are You?" or the nursery rhyme that begins

As I walked by myself
And talked to myself
Myself said unto me,
Look to thyself,

Take care of thyself
For nobody cares for thee.

In long-term situations, the facilitator will find it possible to deliberately pace the rate at which group building and climate-oriented issues are introduced and dealt with. But in short-term bibliotherapy groups, the bibliotherapist may have to open up sensitive issues affecting cohesion and trust both directly and quickly (La Ferriere and Colysen 1978).

Grim themes, however, should not be used in the first few sessions of a bibliotherapy series. In addition to gauging empathically which themes are tolerable for the individual participants to examine at a given time, the facilitator must recognize that the participants need to build up a sense of familiarity both with the bibliotherapist and with the other group members before they will be ready to deal constructively with negative realities.

An extreme example might help to clarify this point. A very idealistic trainee was beginning work with a group of out-patients from a mental hospital who were living in the community. Early on, she decided that her selection of a poem about the dangers of living alone would indicate her sympathetic understanding of the difficulties of their lives. Her choice, "A Sad Song About Greenwich Village," by Frances Park, is certainly a poignant poem. It tells of a woman who lives in a garret with a haunted stair. Each verse concludes with the refrain, "There's nobody . . . to care; . . . to tell; . . . to hear." The last line tells us that even if the woman dies, there is no one who will know. The poem presents a very strong image of an occurrence that, unfortunately, could very well actually happen.

Luckily, the trainee proposed this poem before she actually used it. Her supervisor pointed out that the group memberes were more likely to see the poem as confirmation of their sense of being trapped in a hopeless situation than as an expression of empathy. At the same time, as the trainee did not know the participants or their everyday realities very well yet, she was quite unaware of the ways in which a person living in a difficult situation could do so with dignity. The supervisor was also able to make the point that the chosen material should not gratify the facilitator's impression that she really understands the people she is working with. Rather, the facilitator should put herself in the position of the participant's reality and judge whether she personally could face such a devastating picture.

In this connection, we should note again that some persons find creative writing very threatening both because they do not believe they can write and because they fear exposing their inner thoughts. Thus, the bibliotherapist should use this strategy sparingly—perhaps only as a brief warm-up or wrap-up technique—until a good group climate is established.

In order to get a clearer sense of what stage of cohesion different members are at, trained bibliotherapists have sometimes used the following technique with developmental or chemical dependency groups. Several times in a series of meetings, at the end of the session, pencils and papers are distributed and members are told, "I'd like you to sketch a picture of the group and put yourself in it. Please label yourself. Use arrows if you want to show the dialogue." The drawings are not used as material for dialogue but, rather, are collected and analyzed to help the facilitator see how perceptions and group consciousness have shifted. Hale (1975) does not use this technique but does indicate how role diagramming can illuminate group functioning.

The mature group

Usually there is a point in a stable and closed group at which group members can be observed to have solved inclusion, power, and dependency struggles and to have come together cohesively. At this point, they may have also come to accept and possibly even like each other and to trust other members as well as the facilitator.

In general, this is the most productive period in the life of a group. Members have become willing and able to recognize, examine, juxtapose, and apply the material and to take part in the dialogue. There is less need for warm-ups designed to improve the group climate, and the bibliotherapist can select material that probes individual needs rather than looking for items that will explore group issues such as cohesion and acceptance. At this point, too, the cohesive, supportive atmosphere makes creative writing not only a viable strategy but often a very effective one as well.

The period of group maturity is usually the most rewarding for both bibliotherapist and participants. But even very good bibliotherapists do not always manage to bring a group to this point. For example, it is difficult to sustain highly productive therapeutic group work when membership is open and fluctuates often. Of course, the dynamics of *any* therapeutic group change regularly in any case. Even the most productive developmental groups will go through different phases. Still, the bibliotherapy group is not meant to be a lifelong process. The facilitator must recognize that members can become overly dependent on the group and that their interactions can fall into a comfortable pattern such that, although the members may enjoy the socialization, they do not confront the more painful or complex areas of growth.

Inevitably the time will come when either an individual stops participating or an entire bibliotherapy group ceases to function. Of course, there is a distinction between premature dropping of membership in the group and termination.

Termination

Although the process of growth is endless, we have seen that bibliotherapy is not a lifelong process. The reasons leading to termination are slightly different for clinical and developmental participants. (1) An individual may terminate membership in a clinical setting because the bibliotherapist and the client feel that the person has successfully used bibliotherapy to resolve pertinent conflicts and to improve self-esteem; he or she is now able to apply what has been learned without the support of the therapist or the group. (2) On the other hand, the treatment team and the facilitator may decide to withdraw a patient from bibliotherapy because the person has shown a marked unwillingness to participate or has been repeatedly disruptive. (3) Alternatively, the termination may come as the result of external circumstances such as a change in treatment plans or therapy schedules. (4) On occasion, an entire clinical group will be discontinued because the participants have reached a plateau in their benefits from the materials and the group. Or (5) the bibliotherapist may decide that the need to extend services to other patients warrants the dropping of one group to establish another.

In developmental groups, the reasons for termination will also vary. An individual (or the group as a whole) may decide that he or she has benefited from bibliotherapy but is now ready to move onto something else. Or external circumstances may make it impractical to continue the group. Finally, some developmental groups are scheduled to run only for a fixed period of time, such as during a school year. In any case, once the decision has been made to terminate, the group should be prepared; that is, both clinical and developmental groups should be told of the final meeting date well in advance. It is particularly important that the date and the reason(s) for termination be thoroughly clarified for those who may have difficulty understanding what they are told. For example, in groups made up of retarded or regressed individuals, the bibliotherapist might write the date of the last meeting on a blackboard or flip chart throughout five or six sessions preceding the final one.

Note that it is not uncommon for institutionalized persons to feel abandoned when the end of a group is announced. However, these persons also often suppress their feelings of loss. In this instance, the bibliotherapist should provide ample opportunities for members to express and explore their feelings about the upcoming change.

Meanwhile, the materials and activities related to the termination should be tailored to the group's interests, life experiences, and needs. Both clinical and developmental group members may want to create some expression of their feelings for other group members and the facilitator. Participants might take some time to use pictures, words, and phrases to make collages that express their thoughts; alternatively, they might write or choose a poem that they can then print on different pieces of colored paper to distribute as cards to others.

Clinical and developmental groups alike might choose to make the last meeting a celebration of the enjoyment of earlier meetings. At this time, the members might exchange materials of their own creation or share simple food and drink. The literature selected for use in the final sessions should allow both the participants and the facilitator to express and explore what it means to have a part of one's life stop or change. But, in general, the facilitator will not find it very helpful to depend on materials that emphasize endings as such. Rather, the facilitator should help members see the growth potential in moving on to another phase. Accordingly, the literature might focus on different ways to say good-bye or suggest how beginnings and endings follow each other. For example, "Pruning Trees" by Po Chu-I talks about cutting off the branches of a tree to see a distant mountain, whereas "We Are Transmitters" by D. H. Lawrence points out that simple things like a loaf of homemade bread or a white, freshly washed handkerchief are a way of transmitting life and continuing on with daily life.

Dropping out

It is unrealistic to expect that every participant will be satisfied with or gain optimal help from bibliotherapy. Inevitably, some members will discontinue membership in bibliotherapy groups. Let us look at some of the main factors that may lead to the dropping out of a member. Something about the facilitator's personality or style, for instance, may make some persons too uncomfortable to benefit from the bibliotherapy group. Personality differences are inevitable, and the facilitator should not be unduly troubled when such a situation occurs. However, if a large number of drop-outs occur over a period of time, the bibliotherapist needs to seriously reevaluate how effectively he or she functions so that changes can be made.

There are a number of possible reasons for which the bibliotherapy procedures themselves can lead to a member dropping out. For example, the nature of the material may be a problem: Some persons will not be able to get over their aversion to poetry; others, particularly those who are functionally illiterate might reject all print media. At the other extreme, individuals suffering from paranoia might have a deep mistrust of audiovisual materials and equipment.

In other cases, the problem will involve the dialogue. Discussion of feelings will make some persons intensely uncomfortable. In addition, some schizophrenic individuals, or even young children, will not be able to sort out the images in the material. For others, specifically those incapable of accommodating themselves to innovations, the prospect of dealing with a variety of materials in new ways is too overwhelming. The bibliotherapist should make every effort to help such participants, but there will be times when they are unable or unwilling to overcome the problem and, instead, decide to drop out of the bibliotherapy group.

Participants may also drop out of a bibliotherapy group because of their dissatisfaction with the issues discussed. In such cases, the bibliotherapist will have to carefully evaluate whether the choice of topics and subject matter are rejected only by particular members or whether the dissatisfaction reflects a real weakness in the process itself. The facilitator needs to examine whether he or she (1) is offering too limited a range of topics and genre; (2) is allowing a subgroup to dominate the choice of materials to the exclusion of others' interests; (3) can identify the specific source of dissatisfaction (i.e., do the choices seem irrelevant to the participant, or do they represent issues that this person is reluctant to confront?); (4) has tried to find more engaging materials. If only one or two participants are unhappy and the rest of the group members are interested and engaged by the topics, it may be in everyone's best interests to have the dissatisfied member leave the group, particularly if the unhappiness is a form of resistance. On the other hand, if the dissatisfaction is general, the bibliotherapist may need supervisory help to become more skilled at selecting effective materials.

Another fundamental source of dissatisfaction may have to do with membership of the group. Research on group behavior indicates that participants often seek to belong to groups because they want to be with certain others (Cartwright and Zander 1960). Developmental groups can capitalize on making bibliotherapy a valued activity by involving persons whose association is considered desirable.

On the other hand, as groups are inevitably made up of subgroups, difficulties can arise from intragroup tensions. Once again, note that the problem here is not one of disagreement among members or groups of members; on the contrary, divergency of opinion is often productive. Rather, it is continued hostility or personal animosity toward an individual or subgroup that will eventually destroy the therapeutic climate. Having one member or another drop out might be the only way to resolve clashes of this kind.

In sum, then, the bibliotherapist should consider several possibilities when evaluating what has actually happened when a participant drops out of a bibliotherapy group. As we have seen, the problem may lie in a perfectly normal mismatch of tastes, personalities, or emphasis. At times, the dropout will signal an aspect of personality or skill that the facilitator needs to work on. Finally, particularly in clinical groups, a person may choose or be advised to drop out because that individual is not willing or able to use bibliotherapy as a means of attaining growth and self-understanding.

At the same time, the clinical bibliotherapist should be especially careful to remember that criminals, individuals with chemical addictions, and emotionally disturbed persons have the same right to enjoy or to reject as do persons in developmental groups. Thus the facilitator must look for perfectly normal reasons for dropping out before deciding that a patient or prisoner's reluctance to continue is a further sign of pathology.

STUDY GUIDE

1. In your own words, concisely identify the growth-producing factors of group dynamics.
2. Synthesize your understanding of these phrases: (a) the group as an agent of change; (b) the bibliotherapist as an agent of change; (c) the literature as an agent of change. In addition to the material in the chapter, you might look for examples in one of the following essays, all of which describe the role played by the bibliotherapeutic material in group dynamics: Buck and Kramer (1974), Hannigan (1954), Lessner (1974), Luber (1978), or Rance and Price (1973).
3. Outline the stages in the life-span of a group.
4. Discuss the differences between dropping out and terminating membership in a group as they pertain to both the facilitator and the individual participant.

PRACTICUM

1. Obtain videocassettes or tapes of a group session; use a bibliotherapy experience if possible. Otherwise attend and tape a meeting of a voluntary organization. Identify specific interactions that (a) contribute to group cohesion or further the dialogue in a productive way and that (b) detract from these goals.
2. Give three examples of bibliotherapeutic materials that seem best suited for each stage in the life-span of a group. Provide an analysis of how and why each selection would be useful at these stages.

FURTHER READINGS

Yalom (1975, 1980, 1983) should be read by everyone interested in understanding group process and dynamics. Knowles and Knowles (1972) provide a succinct digest of group dynamics. Garvin (1981) offers a very good analysis of the group processes; pages 85–222 are particularly relevant to the beginnings, working stage, and endings of group life, as well as to the change process. Gruen (1977) also discusses the stages in group life. *Group* and *Group Psychotherapy, Psychodrama and Sociometry* are two periodicals that treat current topics in group theory, whereas Pfeiffer and Jones, and Jones and Pfeiffer issue annual handbooks that catalogue techniques for developing social and facilitory skills, many of which can be adapted to bibliotherapy.

Rosenbaum and Berger (1975) offer essays on different aspects and theories of group functions in therapy groups; the individual authors include Berger, DeRosis, Corsini, Dreikurs, Friedman, and Rosenbaum. Keltner (1973) discusses the interpersonal communications that take place within and outside of groups. Among the chapters that might be useful to bibliotherapists are those dealing with feedback (pages 83–102); nonverbal communication (pages 103–123); and changing behaviors (pages 193–219). Zander (1982) provides a good text on group management. Finally, consult Chapter 12 in Johnson and Johnson (1982) on growth groups.

AFTERWORD

LET US END AS WE BEGAN. But this time we will share some of our reflections on this simple tale that says so much about bibliotherapy.

> *In Cracow, a rabbi dreamt three times that an angel told him to go to Livovna, and that in front of the palace there, near a bridge, he would find a treasure.*

It says here that the rabbi's home is in Cracow and that he goes to Livovna. But it does not really matter where the story takes place—only that the person seeking the treasure of self-knowledge has a home and goes out from it. The cliché is that home is where the heart is—and there is something in that; but this story is telling us that we must go out from ourselves. The literature and the dialogue are like Livovna: They offer us somewhere to go outside of ourselves—some place with a bridge. Indeed, bibliotherapy helps us build a bridge between our cognitive understanding and our feeling-responses.

The story also mentions a rabbi and an angel—appropriately enough. It is not that bibliotherapy has any connection with religion—certainly it is independent of any dogma. But it is a *spiritual* process in the root sense of the word: It is an activity of the human spirit.

> *When the rabbi arrived in Livovna, he told his story to a sentinel who told him that he, too, had had a dream in which he was told to go to a rabbi's house in Cracow, where the treasure was buried in front of the fireplace.*

Sentinel is a rather uncommon word. The translation might have used *guard*, but I like *sentinel* as it somehow better suggests someone who keeps watch or watches over. Yes, the sentinel in this story acts like the bibliotherapist who keeps watch over the dialogue and helps guide participants to the treasure that is buried in front of their own hearths. In fact, the guiding in this story takes place in an exchange between the rabbi and the sentinel about a dream that they shared—just as the bibliotherapist and the participant dialogue about the shared material.

> *So the rabbi went home and dug at his fireplace and found the treasure.*

Everything in this conclusion makes sense in relation to bibliotherapy. The sentinel gave the clue, but it is the rabbi who must act if the treasure is to be found. The bibliotherapist can point the way, but growth is inevitably a personal process. No matter how often someone tells me something about my behavior and attitudes, it is only when I acknowledge the reality to myself that any change in self-understanding occurs.

It is interesting that the story does not specify what was buried in front of the fireplace. But there is a lot to be said for naming one's own treasure. In terms of bibliotherapy, the analogy is obvious: The treasure in front of each hearth may vary from one person to the next, but it is always more precious than gold or diamonds—it is the priceless gift of self-understanding. No material prize could be as valuable, for this spiritual treasure is inexhaustible. As long as we are willing to dig a little deeper, we will continue to reap the benefits.

Appendix A
Listening Exercises

General Directions

As you do these exercises, remember that they pertain to the tool of bibliotherapy but that they do not use the material bibliotherapeutically. The emphasis is on what you and your partner hear in relation to the *content* of the material and the manner of delivery. Before beginning, you may want to review the discussion of the rationale for these exercises in Chapter 1.

- Plan to spend about an hour on each of these exercises (in addition to the time spent selecting items for use). Do not spend more than ten minutes on each evaluation in Exercises 1–3. Also plan to do one exercise as part of the study time scheduled for each of the first six chapters. You will not be able to sustain the kind of concentration necessary for much more than an hour at a time. Then again, skills are best learned when they are exercised repeatedly.
- Make provisions for taping or videotaping the exercises.
- Plan who your listening partner will be; that is, find someone you trust and with whom you can meet conveniently.
- Keep a record of the time spent on this activity, and make notes on your own reactions to your performance. These exercises are part of your training.

Exercise 1

Preparation

Each listening partner (A and B) chooses two brief factual newspaper articles or news summaries of events (200–500 words).

Procedure

Part 1

1. Person A reads the first item aloud, without sharing a copy of the text with person B; then, B orally reports back on what the article was about.

2. Together A and B briefly evaluate how accurately the information was absorbed and reported back. For example, did the report include the five W's of good journalism—Who, What, Where, Why, and When? Consider the different factors affecting the communication, such as how helpful it might have been to have seen a copy of the material.

3. A and B now reverse roles such that B reads the first item selected by B, and A listens and then reports.

4. Again, briefly evaluate A's response, using the points already indicated.

Part 2

While the experience is fresh, use the second article selected by each partner, and repeat steps 1 to 4. This time, however, have B go first and share the text of the article during the reading.

Part 3

1. Analyze what you learned about yourself in doing this exercise. How would you evaluate your partner's performance? What did you learn about recounting the facts of a news story?

2. Make a brief entry in your personal records about how you did on these exercises, and keep the tapes you have made for Exercise 4.

Exercise 2

Preparation

Each partner (A and B) chooses two short short stories (i.e., stories of one page in length) for use in this exercise. Note that some popular magazines regularly feature this kind of story. A human-interest story might also be used, but the emphasis must be on experience rather than facts as such.

Procedure

Part 1

1. Proceed as in Exercise 1: A reads the story; B bases a report on listening only; and both partners evaluate how accurately the sense of the story was absorbed and reported. Again, consider contributing factors, such as how helpful a copy of the text might be. Remember that a short story usually has a discernible beginning, middle, and end. Moreover, it often presents some kind of conflict that needs a solution, or it may end with a purposeful ambiguity. The emphasis is on experience rather than facts.

2. Reverse roles so that B has an opportunity to read an item and A to report. Again, both A and B evaluate the accuracy with which the information was absorbed and reported back.

Part 2

Repeat the process, using the second short short story. As in Exercise 1, have B begin this time and share a copy of the text.

Part 3

Evaluate your performance and that of your partner. What did you learn about recounting the essence of a *story*? Record your observations in your records, and keep your tapes for Exercise 5.

Exercise 3

Preparation

Each listening partner (A and B) selects two poems, one somewhat longer than the other. Avoid using haiku as they are extremely compressed and intentionally ambiguous. As such, they offer less opportunity to test the listener's ability to report content.

Procedure

Part 1

1. Proceed as before: A reads the shorter poem first; B listens and then reports on the ideas, imagery, symbolism or experience depicted in the poem. Note that you are *not* giving a feeling-response at this time; rather, you are concentrating on reporting content. Then briefly evaluate together how well the sense of poem came through; consider factors affecting communication, including the nature of poetry (as compared to articles or stories) and the difficulties posed by not having a copy of the text.
2. Reverse roles, with B reading the shorter poem and A reporting. Again, evaluate the accuracy of the report for about ten minutes.

Part 2

Repeat the procedure with the longer poem. Again, have B read first.

Part 3

Analyze your performance and that of your partner. What did you learn about recounting the essence of a poem? Was there any difference between the poems of different length in terms of the accuracy of the report? Record your observations, and keep your tapes for Exercise 6.

TABLE A.1 Observations

1. Manner of retelling

_____ too much detail so point of message is lost
_____ too little detail to understand the point
_____ haphazardly retells so point is lost
_____ personalizes points so objective content is lost
_____ other (specify) ____________________

2. Accurate listening (evaluate on the basis of how the item was retold)

What does the retelling indicate the reporter was able to hear most accurately?

_____ details about factual matters
_____ details about opinions expressed in the material
_____ details about the story line or intellectual concept
_____ other (specify) ____________________

3. Body language while retelling (more than one item may apply)

_____ aggressive
_____ taciturn
_____ self-confident
_____ tentative
_____ mumbling
_____ comfortable
_____ made eye contact or showed other awareness of listener
_____ nonverbals expressed tension
_____ verbals and nonverbals compatible
_____ verbals and nonverbals incompatible
_____ showed a natural discomfort with a new process
_____ other (specify) ____________________

4. Briefly indicate tone of voice used; note any personal response to the material and the extent to which the response affected the accuracy of reporting about content

____
____
____
____
____

5. Reading ability

_____ reads too fast
_____ reads too slow
_____ reads well (clear voice and diction)
_____ nonverbals seem to express anxiety
_____ other (specify) ____________________

This chart for recording observations about listening skills will be used in Exercises 4, 5, and 6, which all require playing back the tape or videotape made in the first session. Points 1 to 4 apply to the way the listening partners <u>report</u> on each item. Point 5 applies to the <u>reading</u>. (Note that each listening partner will evaluate self and the other for each point. You will probably find it more productive if you observe and discuss each person's performance separately.)

Exercise 4

1. Listen carefully to the tapes made during Exercise 1, and record your observations on Table A.1 for person A's (a) reading ability, and (b) reporting ability.

2. Discuss together any differences between the observations you made when the reading and reporting were done originally and what you see now as you review the tapes. Use the notes you made in the earlier session.

3. Follow the same procedure for person B.

4. Can you make any concrete suggestions to each other regarding techniques for more effective listening and reporting of news stories and factual materials? What might you do differently now that you have had more experience listening to and reporting on different kinds of material?

5. Summarize and record in your notebook your conclusions about the listening efforts involved in comprehending and recounting straight factual material.

Exercise 5

1. Using the tapes you made during Exercise 2, listen and record your observations of both listening partners as you did in Exercise 4.

2. For each partner discuss how your listening skills differed when you used a short short story instead of a news story. Identify the added dimensions that need to be pointed out for clarifying a story as opposed to factual material.

3. Summarize and record in your notebooks your present conclusions about the listening efforts involved in comprehending and recounting short stories. Indicate how your observations changed from the time you first performed the exercise.

Exercise 6

1. Using the tapes made during Exercise 3 and Table A.1, note your observations of both listening partners.

2. Discuss your observations of each partner. Include some analysis of any factor revealed during your review of the session that may have been missed in the original experience. To what extent do these differences indicate greater skill in listening?

3. Note in particular how listening for the content of a poem is different than listening to a news story or a short story. What have your experiences taught you about the nature of the different genres?

4. Summarize and record in your notebook your present conclusions about the listening efforts involved in comprehending and recounting poetry content.

Appendix B
Bibliotherapists' Records

CHRONOLOGICAL RECORD OF BIBLIOTHERAPY SESSIONS CONDUCTED

NAME:

Date	Place	Session	MATERIALS USED: author, title, genre, realia	Supervisor, members, number, type	Audio/ video-tapes	Report written	Cotherapist

REPORT ON BIBLIOTHERAPY GROUP

Trainee's Name______________________________ Division or Ward__________________

Date__________________________

ATTENDANCE: List names in columns followed by a number total.

LITERATURE: Note title and author (attach copy to reports).

COMPLEMENTARY MATERIALS: Music (list selection); other realia (list).

GOALS: For literature and/or group.

REPORT ON THE GROUP: This part should be as objective as possible.

Record what happened in chronological order, including any significant events before or after the group meeting.

Show how the literary tool was used and developed.

Note your interventions and members' responses.

Note nonverbal as well as verbal responses and when members enter or leave room.

EVALUATION AND CRITIQUE:

Record your personal feeling-response.

Record observations of group process, group as a whole, and individuals.

Record trend discussion took and what kind of interventions led to a certain response.

How did your choice of literature or props work?

What additions or changes might you have made?

From your observation, what needs or themes would be helpful in future groups?

NOTE: These reports will provide you and the Bibliotherapy Training Staff with a record of your group. In addition to supplying a learning tool for you, they will provide information from which to develop individual progress notes for patients.

PARTICIPANT'S EVALUATION OF THE BIBLIOTHERAPY EXPERIENCE

The sessions met my expectations. ____________
The sessions did not meet my expectations. ____________

I wish we ____

____

instead of ____

____

The material used
- seemed OK ____________
- related to issues I care about ____________
- helped me learn something about myself ____________
- helped me learn something about how others see me ____________
- did not help me learn anything useful ____________
- was boring ____________
- was irritating because ______________________________

The meeting time was convenient ____________
The meeting would be better attended if held ______________ (day of week)
at ______________ (hour of the day) ______________ (frequency)

The facilitator
- encouraged us to be open and honest ____________
- listened to each of us ____________
- managed the group so we all were heard ____________
- helped us think for ourselves ____________
- talked too much ____________
- bossed us around ____________
- gave too many personal opinions and/or experiences ____________
- always remained in control, never sharing personal things ____________
- asked too many personal questions ____________
- let things go so the sessions were disorderly ____________

Other comments: ____

____

____

On the whole, my reaction to this activity was ______________________________

____

____

ANSWER THE FOLLOWING QUESTIONS ONLY IF YOU CHOOSE:

I feel I have learned ____

____ about myself

I feel my strengths to be ____

____

All in all, I find I have more respect for myself than I did ____________

All in all, I like myself less well than I did, because ______________________

____

The most interesting thing I discovered was ______________________________

____ INITIALS ____________

EVALUATION OF INTERACTIVE PROCESSES

For use by a supervisor, in person or with video or audio tapes. If no supervisor is available, the evaluation can be done by the trainee immediately after filling out the participants' charts.

Name of facilitator________________________ Evaluator________________________

FACILITATOR-INITIATED INTERACTIONS

1. Introduces materials with an intellectual analysis _____

2. Introduces materials briefly; only essentials _____

3. Gives directions: (a) broad gauged _____ (b) very specific _____

4. Asks very narrow, specific questions (to clarify) _____

5. Asks open-ended questions (to encourage) _____

6. Makes interventions by encouraging members: (a) by helpful exploration of feelings _____ (b) by helpful exploration of cognitive reactions _____ (c) by integrating (a) and (b) above _____

7. Also makes interventions by: (a) appropriately letting member(s) take initiative _____ (b) allowing member(s) to "take over" _____ (c) dominating members with talk of self _____ (d) giving advice too frequently or inappropriately _____ (e) cutting off member(s) _____

8. Encourages helpful self-disclosure of member(s) _____

9. Makes self-disclosures that (a) encourage participant(s) _____ (b) answer facilitator's personal needs _____

10. Uses silence: (a) dynamically _____ (b) fears it _____

11. Uses nonverbals to: (a) encourage participants to respond or to continue _____ (b) discourage participants from responding or continuing _____ (c) show respect _____ (d) indicate boredom or indifference _____

12. Establishes climate and boundaries: (a) comfortably _____ (b) erratically, because not agreed upon _____ or because not held to agreed-upon criteria _____

13. Chooses bibliotherapeutic materials that (a) seem appropriate _____ (b) are too volatile, dismaying member(s) _____ (c) do not elicit goal-oriented responses _____

14. Uses complementary material: (a) effectively _____ (b) so that it dominates the session _____ (c) awkwardly, so that it seems to lack relevance _____

FACILITATOR ACCEPTS RESPONSES OF MEMBERS

(Use a through f to record facilitator's reactions.)

Participant's responses		Facilitator's reactions
1. Ideas	_____	(a) clarifies
2. Feelings	_____	(b) reflects
3. Plans for action	_____	(c) encourages
4. Awareness of problems	_____	(d) summarizes
5. Awareness of strengths	_____	(e) comments without rejection
		(f) picks up on later

FACILITATOR REJECTS RESPONSES OF MEMBERS

(Use a through f to record facilitator's reactions.)

Participant's responses		Facilitator's reactions
1. Ideas	_____	(a) invites member(s) evaluation
2. Feelings	_____	(b) only after empathic introduction
3. Plans for action	_____	(c) respectfully gives reasons
4. Awareness of problems	_____	(d) refers back to an earlier remark
5. Awareness of strengths	_____	(e) with little explanation
		(f) brusquely

SUPERVISION FOR TRAINEES

Bibliotherapy supervision focuses on:

1. Guidance in the choice of appropriate and effective literature for the specific group members' needs.

2. Identification of the trainee's personal characteristics and attitudes as they affect the individual and the group discussion.

3. Information and guidance given on the variety of techniques used in the handling of the literature or in the writings of the group members.

4. Information and guidance given on the value and use of complementary materials used to highlight the cognitive and emotional response to the literature.

5. Guidance in identifying and utilizing facilitating interventions on the part of the bibliotherapy trainee.

6. Guidance in identifying and utilizing group discussion to clarify or modify one person's awareness.

7. Guidance in helping the trainee utilize interactions when they are necessary for growth and for handling them when they have become a means of resistance or withdrawal.

8. Helping the trainee observe and utilize group process, especially as it relates to the utilization of the literature as a tool for individual growth.

Appendix C

Professional Organizations

The National Federation for Biblio/Poetry Therapy
Deborah Langosch, ACSW, Executive Secretary
255 Lincoln Place, 2F, Brooklyn, NY 11217
Not-for-profit, invitational membership. Annual meeting.
Established to set and maintain professional standards.

Other Not-for-profit Organizations

American Academy for Poetry Therapy
Morris R. Morrison, Ph.D., Pres.
Suite 424, 255 Congress, Austin, TX 78701

- Training Institute.
- Letter of record of attendance.

Bibliotherapy Forum of the Association of Specialized and Cooperative Library Agencies, a division of the American Library Association.
c/o ALA, 50 E. Huron St., Chicago, IL 60611.
$5.00 a year for ALA members; $7.00 for others interested in membership in the Forum.

- Membership organization.
- Meets twice annually: at the American Library Association Mid-Year and Annual Conventions.
- Newsletter and directory.

Bibliotherapy Round Table
c/o Arleen Hynes, OSB, Pres.
St. Benedict's, St. Joseph, MN 56374

- Not open to membership.
- Offers workshops, courses, and supervisory evaluations. Offers letter of attendance.

Institute for the Study of Bibliotherapy, Inc.
Sister Miriam Schultheis, OSB, Ph.D., Pres.

1671 Spy Run, Fort Wayne, IN 46808.

- Not open to membership.
- Engages in reading education using bibliotherapy.

National Association for Poetry Therapy
Membership to Beverly Harris Bussolati,
1029 Henhawk Rd., Baldwin, NY 11510.
$20.00 a year.

- Membership organization.
- After evaluation offers a CPT (Certified Poetry Therapist).
- Annual meeting. Newsletter.

Poetry Therapy Institute
Arthur Lerner, Ph.D., Pres.
P.O. Box 702, Los Angeles, CA 90070.

- Not open to membership.
- Training institute; letter of record of attendance.
- Offers courses and workshops.

Ohio Poetry Therapy Center and Library
Jennifer Welch
2384 Hardestry Drive So., Columbus, OH 43204

- A regional group that holds workshops and discussions.
- Write for more information.

Bibliography of Professional Literature

Allen, B. 1981a. "Bibliotherapy and the Disabled." *Drexel Library Quarterly* 16.2 (April):81–93.

———. 1981b. *A Guide to Bibliotherapy*, ASCLA Resource List #3. Chicago: American Library Association.

Allen, B., and O'Dell, L. 1981. *Bibliotherapy and the Public Library: The San Rafael Experience*. San Rafael, CA: San Rafael Public Library.

Allen, L., ed. 1981. *Deep Down Things: A Guide for Writing Your Life Story*. Salem, OR: Chemeketa Community College.

Allport, G. W. 1937. *Personality: A Psychological Interpretation*. New York: Holt, Rinehart & Winston.

———. 1950. "A Psychological Approach to the Study of Love and Hate." In *Explorations in Altruistic Love and Hate*, ed. P. Sorokin. Boston: Beacon Press (Kraus Reprint, 1970).

———. 1955. *Becoming: Basic Considerations for a Psychology of Personality*. New Haven: Yale University Press.

Applebaum, S. A. 1966. "Speaking with the Second Voice: Evocativeness." *Journal of the American Psychoanalytic Association* 14.3:402–477.

Applebee, A. N. 1978. *The Child's Concept of Story*. Chicago: University of Chicago Press.

Arbuthnot, M. H., and Sutherland, Z. 1976. *Children and Books*. Glenview, IL: Scott, Foresman & Co.

Arieti, S. 1950. "New Views on the Psychology and Psychopathology of Wit and Comic." *Psychiatry* 13:43–62.

———. 1966. "Creativity and Its Cultivation: Relation to Psychopathology." In *American Handbook of Psychiatry*, vol. 3, ed. S. Arieti. New York: Basic Books.

———. 1967. *The Intrapsychic Self: Feeling, Cognition, and Creativity in Health and Mental Illness*. New York: Basic Books.

———. 1978. "From Primary Process to Creativity." *Journal of Creative Behavior* 12.4:225–246.

Armstrong, B. 1979. "The Creative Arts Therapists: Struggling for Recognition." *Hospital and Community Psychiatry* 30.12 (December):845–847.

Austin, J. H., ed. 1978. *Chase, Chance and Creativity: The Lucky Art of Novelty*. New York: Columbia University Press.

Baldwin, C. 1977. *One to One: Self-understanding Through Journal Writing*. New York: A. Evans & Co.

Baldwin, N. 1976. "The Therapeutic Implications of Poetry Writing: A Methodology." *Journal of Psychedelic Drugs* 8.4 (October–December):307–312.

Ballard, J. 1982. *Stop a Moment: A Group Leader's Handbook of Energizing Experiences.* New York: Irvington.

Bandler, R., and Grinder, J. 1975. *The Structure of Magic: A Book About Language and Therapy,* vol. 1. Palo Alto, CA: Science & Behavior.

Banville, T. G. 1978. *How to Listen—How to Be Heard.* Chicago: Nelson-Hall.

Baruth, L. G., and Phillips, M. W. 1976. "Bibliotherapy and the School Counselor: With Reading Lists for Middleschool Students." *School Counselor* 23 (January):191–199.

Bateson, G. 1979. *Mind and Nature: A Necessary Unity.* New York: Dutton.

Batson, T. W., and Berfman, E., eds. 1976. *The Deaf Experience.* 2d ed. Springfield, MA: Merriam-Eddy.

Beatty, W. K. 1962. "A Historical Review of Bibliotherapy." *Library Trends* 11 (October):106–117.

Beck, A. P. 1974. "Phases in the Development of Structure in Therapy and Encounter Groups." *Innovations in Client-centered Therapy,* pp. 441–464. New York: Wiley.

Bell, G. 1982. "Poetry Therapy: Changing Concepts and Emerging Questions." *Arts in Psychotherapy* 9.1 (Spring):25–30.

Benninger, J., and Belli, E. 1982. "Social Development in the Classroom." *Viewpoints in Teaching and Learning* 58.1 (Winter):128–131.

Berchter, H. J. 1979. *Group Participation: Techniques for Leaders and Members.* Beverly Hills, CA: Sage.

Berchter, H. J., and Maple, F. F. 1977. *Creating Groups.* Beverly Hills, CA: Sage.

Berg-Cross, G., and Berg-Cross, L. 1976. "Bibliotherapy for Young Children." *Journal of Clinical Child Psychology* 5.2 (Fall):35–38, 70.

Berger, M. 1975. "Nonverbal Communications in Group Psychotherapy." In *Group Psychotherapy and Group Function,* rev. ed., ed. M. Rosenbaum and M. Berger. New York: Basic Books.

______. 1978. *Videotape Techniques in Psychiatric Training and Treatment.* 2d ed. New York: Basic Books.

Berger, M., and Rosenbaum, M. 1967. "Notes on Help-rejecting Complainers." *International Journal of Group Psychotherapy* 17:357–370.

Bernstein, B. 1981. "Psychiatric Therapy Through the Creative Arts." *Journal of Creative Behaviors* 15.3:103–108.

Berry, F. M. 1977. "Analysis of Process in Bibliotherapy." In "Proceedings of the Fourth Bibliotherapy Round Table," ed. A. Hynes and K. Gorelick, pp. 25–37. Washington, DC.

Bettleheim, B. 1976. *The Uses of Enchantment: The Meaning and Importance of Fairy Tales.* New York: Knopf.

Bion, W. R. 1961. *Experience in Groups.* New York: Ballantine.

Blanton, S. 1960. *The Healing Power of Poetry.* New York: Thomas Y. Crowell.

Bleich, D. 1975. *Readings and Feelings: An Introduction to Subjective Criticism.* Urbana, IL: National Council of Teachers of English.

Borriello, J. F. 1973. "Patients with Acting-out Character Disorders." *American Journal of Psychotherapy* 27:4–14.

______. 1976. "Group Psychotherapy in Hospital Systems." In *Group Therapy,* eds. A. Walberg and M. Aronson. New York: Stratton Intercon.

Bowker, M. A. 1982. "Children and Divorce: Being in Between." *Elementary School Guidance* 17.2:126–130.

Bracken, J., and Wigotoff, S. 1979. *Books for Today's Children.* Old Westbury, NY: Feminist Press.

Branden, N. 1969. *The Psychology of Self-esteem: A New Concept of Man's Psychological Nature.* Los Angeles: Nash.

Bresler, E. 1981. "The Use of Poetry Therapy with Older People." *Aging* (January-February):23–27.

Brown, D. H. 1977. "Poetry as a Counseling Tool: The Relationship Between Responses to Emotion-oriented Poetry and Emotions, Interests, and Personal Needs." Ph.D. thesis, Cornell University.

Brown, E. F. 1975. *Bibliotherapy and Its Widening Applications.* Metuchen, NJ: Scarecrow.

Brown, R. M. 1977. "Bibliotherapy as a Technique for Increasing Individuality Among Elderly Patients." *Hospital and Community Psychiatry* 28.5 (May):347.

Bryan, A. I. 1939. "Can There Be a Science of Bibliotherapy?" *Library Journal* 64 (October):773–776.

Buber, M. 1963. "Healing Through Meeting." In *Pointing the Way: Collected Essays by Martin Buber*, ed. M. Buber. New York: Harper & Row.

______. 1970. *I and Thou*. New York: Scribner.

Buck, L. A., and Kramer, A. 1973. "Opening New Worlds to the Deaf and Disturbed." In *Poetry the Healer*, ed. J. J. Leedy. Philadelphia: Lippincott.

______. 1974. "Poetry as a Means of Group Facilitation." *Journal of Humanistic Psychology* 14.1 (Winter):65–71.

Burns, M. 1977. "Poetry Therapy: A Tool to Foster Creativity." *Art Psychotherapy* 4.2:95–98.

Burnside, I. M., ed. 1983. *Working with the Elderly: Group Processes and Techniques*, 2d ed. Los Angeles: Wadsworth.

Burt, L. 1972. "Bibliotherapy: Effects of Group Reading and Discussion on Attitudes of Adult Inmates in Two Correctional Institutions." Ph.D. thesis, University of Wisconsin, Madison.

Butler, R. 1977. *Aging and Mental Health: Positive Psychosocial Approaches*. St. Louis: Mosby.

Butterfield-Picard, H., et al. 1982. "Hospice the Adjective, Not the Noun: The Future of a National Priority." *American Psychology* 37.11:1254–1259.

Cacha, F. B. 1978. "Book Therapy for Abused Children." *Language Arts* 55 (February):199–202.

Campbell, J. 1976. *The Masks of God: Creative Mythology*. New York: Penguin.

Carkhuff, R. 1969. *Helping and Human Relations: A Primer for Lay and Professional Helpers*, vol. 1. New York: Holt, Rinehart & Winston.

______. 1983. *The Art of Helping*, 5th ed. Amherst, MA: Human Resources Development Press.

Cartwright, D., and Zander, T. 1960. *Group Dynamics Research and Theory*, 2d ed. Evanston, IL: Row, Peterson & Co.

Cellini, H. R., and Young, O. 1976. "Bibliotherapy in Institutions." *Transactional Analysis Journal* 6.4 (October):407–409.

Chambers, D. W. 1977. *The Oral Tradition: Storytelling and Creative Drama*, 2d ed. Dubuque: Brown.

Chavis, G. 1984. "Poetry Therapy in a Women's Growth Group on the Mother-Daughter Connection" (address given at the Fourth National Poetry Association Meeting, April, Hempstead, NY).

Chevin, R., and Neill, M. 1980. *The Woman's Tale: A Journal of Inner Exploration*. New York: Crossroad Books Seabury.

Clancy, M., and Lauer, R. 1978. "Zen Telegrams: A Warm-up Technique for Poetry Therapy Groups." In *Poetry in the Therapeutic Experience*, ed. A. Lerner. New York: Pergamon.

Combs, A. W. 1978. *Helping Relationships: Basic Concepts for the Helping Professions*, 2d ed. Rockleigh, NJ: Allyn.

Compton, M., and Skelton, J. 1982. "A Study of Selected Adolescent Problems as Presented in Contemporary Realistic Fiction for Middle School Students." *Adolescence* 17.67:637–645.

Corsini, R. J., and Rosenberg, B. 1975. "Mechanisms of Group Psychotherapy Processes and Dynamics." In *Group Psychotherapy and Group Functions*, rev. ed., ed. M. Rosenbaum and M. Berger. New York: Basic Books.

Cousins, N. 1979. *Anatomy of an Illness as Perceived by the Patient*. New York: Norton.

Cox, H. 1969. *The Feast of Fools: A Theological Essay on Festivity and Fantasy*. Cambridge, MA: Harvard University Press.

Crootof, C. 1969. "Poetry Therapy for Psychoneurotics in a Mental Health Center." In *Poetry Therapy*, ed. J. J. Leedy. Philadelphia: Lippincott.

Crosson, J. D. 1975. *The Dark Interval: Towards a Theology of Story*. Niles, IL: Argus Communications.

Danish, S. J., et al. 1980. *Helping Skills: A Basic Training Program*, 2d ed. (Trainee's Workbook). New York: Human Sciences Press.

D'Augelli, A. R., et al. 1980. *Helping Skills: A Basic Training Program*, 2d ed. (Leader's Manual). New York: Human Sciences Press.

De Rosis, H. 1975. "Karen Horney's Theory Applied to Psychoanalysis in Groups." In *Group Psychotherapy and Group Function*, rev. ed., ed. M. Rosenbaum and M. Berger. New York: Basic Books.

______. 1978. *Working with Patients: Introductory Guidelines for Psychotherapists.* New York: Agathon.

Deutsch, H. 1973. *Confrontations with Myself: An Epilogue*. New York: Norton.

Dillard, J. M. 1983. *Multicultural Counseling*. New York: Nelson-Hall.

Dreikurs, R. 1975. "Group Psychotherapy from the Point of View of Adlerian Psychology." In *Group Psychotherapy and Group Function*, rev. ed., ed. M. Rosenbaum and M. Berger. New York: Basic Books.

DSM III. 1980. *Diagnostic and Statistical Manual of Mental Disorders*, 3d ed. Washington, DC: American Psychiatric Association.

Duschesne, L. 1950. "The Factors of Altruism." In *Explorations in Altruistic Love and Behavior*, ed. P. Sorokin. Boston: Beacon Press (Kraus Reprint, 1970).

Edgar, K. 1978. "The Epiphany of the Self Via Poetry Therapy." In *Poetry in the Therapeutic Experience*, ed. A. Lerner. New York: Pergamon.

______. 1979. "A Case of Poetry Therapy." *Psychotherapy: Theory, Research and Practice* 16.1 (Spring):104–106.

Edgar, K., and Hazley, R. 1969. "Validation of Poetry Therapy as a Group Therapy Technique." In *Poetry Therapy*, ed. J. J. Leedy. Philadelphia: Lippincott.

Edgar, K., Hazley, R., and Levitt, H. 1969. "Poetry Therapy with Hospitalized Schizophrenics." In *Poetry the Healer*, ed. J. J. Leedy. Philadelphia: Lippincott.

Egan, G. 1975. *The Skilled Helper: A Model for Systematic Helping and Interpersonal Relating*. Monterey, CA: Brooks-Cole.

Ekman, P., ed. 1972. *Emotion in the Human Face*. New York: Pergamon.

Elias, M. J. 1983. "Improving Coping Skills of Emotionally Disturbed Boys Through T.V. Social Problem Solving." *American Journal of Orthopsychiatry* 53.1 (January):61–72.

Elkins, D. P., ed. 1979. *Self-concept Sourcebook: Ideas and Activities for Building Self-esteem*. Rochester, NY: Growth Association.

Ellis, A. 1969. "Rational-Emotive Therapy." *Journal of Continuing Psychotherapy* 1.2:82–90.

Erikson, E. 1964. *Insight and Responsibility.* New York: Norton.

Esler, H. 1982. "Bibliotherapy in Practice." *Library Trends* (Spring):647–659.

Ewens, J., and Harrington, P. 1982. *Hospice: A Handbook for Families and Others Facing Terminal Illness.* Santa Fe: Bear and Co.

Favazza, A. R. 1966. "Bibliotherapy: A Critique of the Literature." *Bulletin of the Medical Library Association* 54.2 (April):138–141.

Fincher, J. 1975. "Dialogue in a Journal." *Human Behavior* (November):17–23.

Fingarette, H. 1963. *The Self in Transformation*. New York: Basic Books.

Fogle, D. M. 1980. "Art and Poetry Therapy Combined with Talking Therapy with a Family of Four in an Outpatient Clinic." *Arts in Psychotherapy* 7.1:27–34.

Forrest, D. 1976. "Nonsense and Sense in Schizophrenic Language." *Schizophrenia Bulletin NIMH* 2.2:286–301.

Frank, J. D. 1968. *Magical Healing and Psychotherapy* (phonotape). New York: McGraw-Hill.

______. 1972. "Common Features Account for Effectiveness." In *Changing Frontiers in the Science of Psychotherapy*, ed. A. Bergin and H. Strump. Chicago: Aldine, Atherton.

______. 1973. *Persuasion and Healing: A Comparative Study of Psychotherapy*, rev. ed. Baltimore: Johns Hopkins University Press.

______. 1974. "Psychotherapy: The Restoration of Morale." *American Journal of Psychiatry* 131.3 (March):271–274.

______. 1978. *Effective Ingredients of Successful Psychotherapy.* New York: Brunner/Mazel.

Frasier, M., and McCannon, C. 1981. "Using Bibliotherapy with Gifted Children." *Gifted Child Quarterly* 25.2 (Spring):81–85.

Freytag, G. 1977. "Services for the Handicapped: Bibliotherapy by Means of Picture Books for Speech-handicapped Children." *International Library Review* 9 (April):197–203.

Friedman, M. 1975. "Dialogue and the 'Essential We': The Bases of Values in the Philosophy of Martin Buber." In *Group Psychotherapy and Group Function*, rev. ed., ed. M. Rosenbaum and M. Berger. New York: Basic Books.

______. 1976. "Healing Through Meeting: A Dialogical Approach to Psychotherapy and Family Therapy." In *Psychiatry and the Humanities,* ed. J. H. Smith. New Haven: Yale University Press.

Fromm, E. 1951. *The Forgotten Language: An Introduction to the Understanding of Dreams, Fairy Tales, and Myths.* New York: Holt, Rinehart & Winston.

______. 1956. *The Art of Loving.* New York: Harper & Row.

Fromm-Reichman, F. 1950. *Principles of Intensive Psychotherapy.* Chicago: University of Psychotherapy Chicago Press.

Frost, R. 1963. "Introduction" to *The Selected Poems of Robert Frost.* New York: Holt, Rinehart & Winston.

Gallagher, T. 1980. "The Poem as Time Machine." *Atlantic Monthly* (May):70–75.

Gardner, R. A. 1969. "Mutual Storytelling as a Technique in Child Psychotherapy and Psychoanalysis." In *Science and Psychoanalysis,* vol. 14, ed. J. Masserman. New York: Grune.

______. 1971. *Therapeutic Communication with Children: The Mutual Storytelling Technique in Child Psychotherapy.* New York: Aronson.

Garvin, C. D. 1981. *Contemporary Group Work.* Englewood Cliffs, NJ: Prentice-Hall.

Gaylin, N. L. 1974. "On Creativeness and a Psychology of Well-being." In *Innovations in Client-centered Therapy,* ed. R. J. Corsini. New York: Wiley.

Gaylin, W. 1979. *Feelings: Our Vital Signs.* New York: Ballantine.

Gendlin, E. T. 1971. "Sub-verbal Communication and Therapist Activity: Trends in Client-centered Therapy with Schizophrenics." In *Person to Person,* ed. C. Rogers and B. Stevens. New York: Pocket Books.

Gladding, S. T. 1979. "The Creative Use of Poetry in the Counseling Process." *Personnel and Guidance Journal* (February):285–287.

______. 1984. The Family Poem. (address given at the Fourth National Poetry Association, Hampstead, NY).

Glasgow, R. E., and Rosen, G. M. 1978. "Behavioral Bibliotherapy: A Review of Self-help Manuals." *Psychological Bulletin* 85.1 (January):1–23.

Goble, F. G. 1971. *The Third Force: The Psychology of Abraham Maslow.* New York: Pocket Books.

Goldfield, M., and Lauer, R. 1971. "The Use of Creative Writing in Young Adult Drug Abusers." *New Physician* 20:449–457.

Goleman, D. 1979. "Positive Denial: The Case for Not Facing Reality (Richard S. Lazarus interviewed by Daniel Goleman)." *Psychology Today* (November):44–60.

Greenbaum, J., et al. 1980. "Using Books About Handicapped Children." *Reading Teacher* 33 (January):416–419.

Greenblatt, M. 1950. "Altruism in the Psychotherapeutic Relationship." In *Explorations in Altruistic Love and Behavior,* ed. P. Sorokin. Boston: Beacon (Kraus Reprint, 1970).

Grinder, J., and Bandler, R. 1976. *The Structure of Magic,* vol. 2. Palo Alto, CA: Science and Behavior.

Gruen, W. 1977. "The Stages in the Development of a Therapy Group: Tell-tale Symptoms and Their Origins in the Dynamic Group Forces." *Group* 1.1 (Spring): 10–17.

Hale, A. E. 1975. "The Role Diagram Expanded." *Group Psychotherapy and Psychodrama* 28:77–103.

Hall, C. S., and Lindzey, G. 1957. *Theories of Personality.* New York: Wiley.

Hall, E. 1976. "How Cultures Collide." *Psychology Today* (July):66–75.

Hallowell, E. M. 1983. "Communication Through Poetry in the Therapy of a Schizophrenic Patient." *Journal of the American Academy of Psychoanalysis* 11.1 (January):133–158.

Hammond, C. D., et al. 1978. *Improving Therapeutic Communication.* San Francisco: Jossey-Bass.

Hannigan, M. C. 1954. "An Experience in Group Bibliotherapy." *ALA Bulletin* (March):148–150.

Harrower, M. 1972. *The Therapy of Poetry.* Springfield, IL: Thomas.

Hastings, A. C., et al. 1980. *Health for the Whole Person: The Complete Guide for Holistic Medicine.* Boulder, CO: Westview Press.

Havens, L. L. 1974. "The Existential Use of the Self." *American Journal of Psychiatry* 131.1 (January):1–10.

Heninger, O. E. 1977. "Poetry Therapy: Exploration of a Creative Writing Maneuver." *Art Psychotherapy* 4:39–40.

______. 1978. "Poetry Therapy in Private Practice: An Odyssey into the Healing Power of Poetry." In *Poetry in the Therapeutic Experience*, ed. A. Lerner. New York: Pergamon.

Heymann, D. A. 1974. "Discussions Meet Needs of Dying Patients." *Hospitals, Journal of American Hospitals Association* (July 16):57–62.

Hinseth, L. 1975. "Contract Considerations in the Practice of Bibliotherapy." *Health and Rehabilitative Library Services* 1.2 (October):21–22.

Hoffman, M. L. 1965. "Empathy: Its Development and Prosocial Implications." In *Nebraska Symposium on Motivation*, vol. 13, ed. B. Keasy. Lincoln: University of Nebraska.

Holland, N. N. 1975. *Five Readers Reading*. New Haven: Yale University Press.

Horney, K. 1945. *Our Inner Conflicts: A Constructive Theory of Neurosis.* New York: Norton.

______. 1950. *Neurosis and Human Growth*. New York: Norton.

Huck, C. 1976. *Children's Literature in Elementary School*, 3d ed. New York: Harper & Row.

Hynes, A. 1975a. "Bibliotherapy at St. Elizabeths Hospital." *Health and Rehabilitative Library Services* 1.2 (October):18–19.

______. 1975b. "Bibliography of Bibliotherapy Reference Materials, 1970–1975." *Health and Rehabilitative Library Services* 1.2 (October):22–25.

______. 1977. "Rationale for a Bibliotherapy Training Program." In "Proceedings of the Fourth Bibliotherapy Round Table," ed. A. Hynes and K. Gorelick. Washington, DC.

______. 1978a. "Certification in the St. Elizabeths Bibliotherapy Training Program." In *Using Bibliotherapy*, ed. R. Rubin. Phoenix, AZ: Oryx Press.

______. 1978b. "Bibliotherapy in the Circulating Library at St. Elizabeths Hospital." *Bibliotherapy Sourcebook*, ed. R. Rubin. Phoenix, AZ: Oryx Press.

______. 1978c. "Education of a Bibliotherapist." In *Seminar on Bibliotherapy: Proceedings*, ed. M. Monroe. Madison: University of Wisconsin Library School.

______. 1979. "Bibliotherapy and the Aging." *Catholic Library World* 50.7 (February):280–284.

Izard, C. 1977. *Human Emotion*. New York: Plenum.

Jacobs, G. H. 1970. *When Children Think: Using Journals to Encourage Creative Thinking.* New York: Teacher's College Press.

Jahoda, M. 1958. *Current Concepts of Positive Mental Health*, Monograph series no. 1. New York: Basic Books.

Jalongo, M. R. 1983a. "Using Crisis-oriented Books with Young Children." *Young Children* (July):29–35.

______. 1983b. "Bibliotherapy: Literature to Promote Socioemotional Growth." *Reading Teacher* (April):796–803.

Jaskoski, H. 1980. "Poetry, Poetics and the Poetry Therapist." *Arts in Psychotherapy* 7.4:75–79.

Johnson, D. W., and Johnson, F. P. 1982. *Joining Together: Group Theory and Group Skills*, 2d ed. Englewood Cliffs, NJ: Prentice-Hall.

Jones, J., and Pfeiffer, J. 1977. *The 1977 Annual Handbook for Group Facilitators.* La Jolla, CA: University Association.

Joseph, S. M. 1969. *The Me Nobody Knows: Children's Voices from the Ghetto.* New York: Avon.

Jourard, S. M. 1964. *The Transparent Self.* Princeton, NJ: Van Nostrand.

Jung, C. G. 1968. "The Archetype and the Collective Unconscious." In *The Collected Works of C. G. Jung*, vol. 9, pt. 1, Princeton, NJ: Princeton University Press.

Kaminsky, M. 1974. *What's Inside You Shines Out of You*. New York: Horizon.

Kanaan, J. 1975. "The Application of Adjuvant Bibliotherapeutic Techniques in Resolving Peer Acceptance Problems." Ed.D. thesis, University of Pittsburgh.

Kaplan, A., and Bean, J. 1976. *Beyond Sex-role Stereotypes: Readings Toward a Psychology of Androgyny.* Boston: Little, Brown.

Keen, S., and Fox, A. V. 1973. *Telling Your Story: A Guide to Who You Are and Who You Can Be.* Garden City, NJ: Doubleday.

Keltner, J. W. 1973. *Elements of Interpersonal Communication*. Belmont, CA: Wadsworth.

Kenny, B. L. 1982. "Audiovisuals in Mental Health." *Library Trends* 30.4 (Spring):591–611.

Kenz, C. A. 1982. "School Librarian as Bibliotherapist." *Catholic Library World* 54:219–221.

Kilguss, A. 1974. "Using Soap Operas as a Therapeutic Tool." *Social Casework* (November):525–530.

Knapp, M. L. 1980. *Essentials of Nonverbal Communication*. New York: Holt, Rinehart & Winston.

Knowles, M., and Knowles, H. 1972. *Introduction to Group Dynamics*. Chicago: Follett.

Kobak, D. 1975. "The Use of Creativity Techniques in the Bereavement of Widows." *Archives of the Foundations of Thanatology* 5.1 (January):48.

Koch, K. 1970. *Wishes, Lies and Dreams*. New York: Chelsea House.

______. 1973. *Rose, Where Did You Get that Red? Teaching Great Poetry to Children*. New York: Random House.

______. 1977. *I Never Told Anybody: Teaching Writing in a Nursing Home*. New York: Random House.

Kochman, T. 1981. *Black and White Styles in Conflict*. Chicago: University of Chicago Press.

Kosinski, L. V. 1968. *Readings in Creativity and Imagination in Literature and Language*. Washington, DC: National Council of Teachers of English.

Kravetz, D., and Jones, L. E. 1981. "Androgyny as a Standard of Mental Health." *American Journal of Orthopsychiatry* 51.3 (July):502–509.

Kubie, L. 1961. *Neurotic Distortion of the Creative Process*. New York: Noonday Press.

Kubler-Ross, E. 1969. *On Death and Dying*. New York: Macmillan.

______. 1975. *Death: The Final Stage of Growth*. Englewood Cliffs, NJ: Prentice-Hall.

______. 1978. *To Live Until We Say Goodbye*. Englewood Cliffs, NJ: Prentice-Hall.

Lack, C. 1978. "Adult Bibliotherapy Discussion Group Bibliography." In *Using Bibliotherapy*, ed. R. Rubin. Phoenix, AZ: Oryx Press.

______. 1982. "Biblio/Poetry Therapy with Acute Patients." *The Arts in Psychotherapy* 9:291–295.

Lack, C., and Bettencourt, B. 1973. "Bibliotherapy in the Community." *News Notes of California Libraries* 67 (Fall):374–376.

La Ferriere, L., and Colysen, R. 1978. "Goal Attainment Scaling: An Effective Treatment Technique in Short-term Therapy." *American Journal of Community Psychology* 6.3:271–282.

Langs, R. 1978. *The Listening Process*. New York: Jacob Aronson, Inc.

Lauer, R. 1972. "Creative Writing as a Therapeutic Tool." *Hospital and Community Psychiatry* 23:39–40.

______. 1978. "Abuses of Poetry Therapy." In *Poetry in the Therapeutic Experience*, ed. A. Lerner. New York: Pergamon.

Lauer, R., and Goldfield, M. 1970. "Creative Writing in Group Therapy." *Psychotherapy: Theory, Research and Practice* 7.4 (Winter):248–251.

Lawrence, N. H. 1978. *Soul's Inner Sparkle: Moments of Waka Sensations*. Tokyo: Eichosha.

Lazarus, R. S. 1966. *Psychological Stress and the Coping Process*. New York: McGraw-Hill.

______. 1974. "Cognitive and Coping Processes in Emotion." In *Cognitive Views of Human Motivation*, ed. B. Weiner. New York: Academic Press.

Leedy, J. J., ed. 1969. *Poetry Therapy: The Use of Poetry in the Treatment of Emotional Disorders*. Philadelphia: Lippincott.

______. 1973. *Poetry the Healer*. Philadelphia: Lippincott.

Lerner, A. 1979. "A Note on Poetry Therapy." *Art Psychotherapy* 6.3:197–198.

______. 1981. "Poetry Therapy." In *Handbook of Innovative Therapies*, ed. R. J. Corsini. New York: Wiley.

______. 1982. "Poetry Therapy in the Group Experience." In *The Newer Therapies: A Sourcebook*, ed. L. Abt and I. Stuart. New York: Van Nostrand Reinhold.

______. 1984a. "Bibliotherapy." In *The Encyclopedia of Psychology*, ed. R. J. Corsini. New York: Wiley.

______. 1984b. "Poetry Therapy." In *The Encyclopedia of Psychology*, ed. R. J. Corsini. New York: Wiley.

Lerner, A., ed. 1978. *Poetry in the Therapeutic Experience*. New York: Pergamon.

Lessner, J. W. 1974. "The Poem as Catalyst in Group Counseling." *Personnel and Guidance Journal* 53 (September):33–38.

Lewis, M. I., and Butler, R. N. 1974. "Life-review Therapy: Putting Memories to Work in Individual and Group Psychotherapy." *Geriatrics* 29:165–174.

Long, L. 1978. *Listening/Responding: Human Relations Training for Teachers.* Belmont, CA: Wadsworth.

Luber, R. F. 1973. "Poetry Helps Patients Express Feelings." *Hospital and Community Psychiatry* 24:284.

______. 1976. "Poetry Therapy: An Introduction to Theory and Technique." In *Proceedings of the Annual Conference on Partial Hospitalization,* ed. R. A. Luber.

______. 1978. "Recurrent Spontaneous Themes in Group Poetry Therapy." *Art Psychotherapy* 5:55–60.

Lundsteen, S. 1964. "A Thinking Improvement Program Through Literature." *Elementary English* (October 6):505–507.

Lynch, W. F. 1965. *Images of Hope: Imagination, Healer of the Hopeless.* New York: Mentor.

MacNamee, G. D. 1985. "The Social Origins of Narrative Skills." In *Social and Functional Approaches to Language and Thought,* ed. Maya Hickman. New York: Academic Press.

Maher, B. 1972. "The Language of Schizophrenia: A Review and Interpretation." *British Journal of Psychiatry* 12:3–17.

Marmor, J. 1975. "The Nature of the Therapeutic Process Revisited." *Canadian Psychiatric Association Journal* 20.8:557–565.

Marshall, M. 1981. *Libraries and the Handicapped Child.* Boulder, CO: Westview Press.

Martin, M., et al. 1983. "Bibliotherapy: Children of Divorce." *School Counselor* 30:312–315.

Maslow, A. H. 1962. *Toward a Psychology of Being.* Princeton: Van Nostrand.

______. 1967. "The Creative Attitude." In *Explorations in Creativity,* ed. L. Mooney and S. Razik. New York: Harper & Row.

______. 1970. *Motivation and Personality.* 2d ed. New York: Harper & Row.

______. 1971a. *The Farther Reaches of Human Behavior.* New York: Allyn & Bacon.

______. 1971b. "The Creative Attitude." In *The Helping Relationship Sourcebook,* ed. D. Avila et al. Boston: Allyn & Bacon.

Maultsby, M. 1984. *Rational Behavior Therapy.* Englewood Cliffs, NJ: Prentice-Hall.

May, R. 1975. *The Courage to Create.* New York: Norton.

Mazza, N. 1979. "Poetry: A Therapeutic Tool in the Early Stages of Alcoholism Treatment." *Journal of Studies on Alcohol* 40.1:123–128.

______. 1981. "The Use of Poetry in Treating the Troubled Adolescent." *Adolescence* 16.62 (Summer):403–408.

Mazza, N., and Prescott, B. 1981. "Poetry: An Ancillary Technique in Couples Group Therapy." *American Journal of Family Therapy* 9.1 (Spring):53–57.

McConnell, F. D. 1979. *Storytelling and Mythology: Images from Film and Literature.* New York: Oxford University Press.

McKay, M. 1978. "Writing and the Schizophrenic Patient." *Cimarron Review* (October):51–57.

McKellar, P. H. 1957. *Imagination and Thinking: A Psychological Analysis.* New York: Basic Books.

McLeish, J.A.B. 1976. *The Ulyssean Adult: Creativity in the Middle and Later Years.* Toronto: McGraw-Hill Ryerson, Ltd.

Meerlo, J.A.M. 1969. "The Universal Language of Rhythm." In *Poetry Therapy,* ed. J. J. Leedy. Philadelphia: Lippincott.

Meichenbaum, D., and Cameron, R. 1974. "The Clinical Potential of Modifying What Clients Say to Themselves." *Psychotherapy: Theory, Research and Practice* 11:103–119.

Meissner, W. W. 1977. "Cognitive Aspects of the Paranoid Process-Prosepectus." In *Thought, Consciousness and Reality,* vol. 2, ed. J. H. Smith. New Haven: Yale University Press.

Merriam, S. 1980. "The Concept and Function of Reminiscence: A Review of the Research." *Gerontologist* 20:604–609.

Meyerowitz, J. H., and Driskill, L. 1975. "Using Narrative Skills in the Rehabilitation of Hospitalized Drug Addicts." *Hospital and Community Psychiatry* 26.6 (January):335–339.

Miller, A. H. 1983. "The Spontaneous Use of Poetry in an Adolescent Girl's Group." *International Journal of Psychotherapy* 23.2:223–237.

Miller, D. K. 1978. "Poetry Therapy with Psychotic Patients." *Journal of Contemporary Psychotherapy* 9.2:135–138.

Miller, J. 1972. *Word, Self, Reality: The Rhetoric of Imagination*. New York: Dodd.
Mitchell, D. 1978. "A Note on Art Psychotherapy and Poetry Therapy: The Coordination of Art and Poetry as an Expressive Technique." *Art Psychotherapy* 5.4:223–225.
Monroe, M., and Rubin, R. 1983. *The Challenge of Aging: A Bibliography.* Littleton, CO: Libraries Unlimited.
Moody, M. 1964. "Bibliotherapy for Chronic Illnesses." *Hospital Progress* 45 (January):62–63.
Moody, M. T., and Limper, H. 1971. *Bibliotherapy: Materials and Methods.* Chicago: American Library Association.
Moody, R. 1978. *Laugh After Laugh.* Newport Beach, CA: Headwaters Press.
Moore, T. V. 1946. "Bibliotherapy in Psychiatric Practice." In *Current Therapies of Personality Disorders,* ed. B. Glueck. New York: Grune.
Morrison, M. 1973. "A Defense of Poetry Therapy." In *Poetry the Healer,* ed. J. J. Leedy. Philadelphia: Lippincott.
______. 1978. "The Use of Poetry in the Treatment of Emotional Dysfunction." *Art Psychotherapy* 5.2:93–98.
Neale, G. 1981. "Poetry and Movement Therapy with an Institutionalized Geriatric Population: Working Through Losses and Consolidating Strengths." *Pratt Institute Creative Arts Therapy Review* 2:25–36.
Nickerson, E. T. 1975. "Bibliotherapy: A Therapeutic Medium for Helping Children." *Psychotherapy: Theory, Research and Practice* 12.3 (Fall):258–261.
Norman, R., and Brockmeier, S. 1979. "Bibliotherapy from Theory to Practice." *Nebraska Library Association Quarterly* 10 (Spring):14–17.
O'Dell, L. 1983. "Bibliotherapy and the Elderly." In *Working with the Elderly: Group Processes and Techniques,* 2d ed., ed. I. Burnside, Belmont CA: Wadsworth.
Otto, H. A. 1963. *The Otto Inventory of Personal Resources* (n.p.).
______. 1965. "Personality Strengths Concept in the Helping Professions." *Psychiatric Quarterly* 39 (October):632–645.
______. 1966. "Adolescents' Self-perception of Personality Strengths." *Journal of Human Relations* 14.3:483–491.
______. 1968a. *Human Potentials: The Challenge and the Promise.* St. Louis: Green.
______. 1968b. *Ways of Growth: Approaches to Expanding Awareness.* New York: Grossman.
______. 1973. *Group Methods to Actualize Human Potential: A Handbook,* 3d limited ed. Beverly Hills, CA: Holistic Press.
______. 1979. *Dimensions in Holistic Healing.* Chicago: Nelson-Hall.
Overstad, B. 1981. *Bibliotherapy: Books to help young children.* St. Paul, MN: Toys 'n Things Press.
Parloff, M. 1969. "Assessing the Effects of Headshrinking and Mind-Expanding" (paper read at the American Group Psychotherapy Association meeting, New York).
Parloff, M., et al. 1978. "Research on Therapist Variables in Relation to Process and Outcome." In *Handbook of Psychotherapy and Behavioral Change: An Empirical Analysis,* 2d ed., ed. S. Garfield and A. Bergin. New York: Wiley.
Parnes, S. J., and Harding, H. F. 1962. *A Sourcebook of Creative Thinking.* New York: Scribner.
Pattison, E. M. 1973. "The Psychodynamics of Poetry by Patients." In *Poetry the Healer,* ed. J. J. Leedy. Philadelphia: Lippincott.
Pearle, D., et al. 1982. *Television and Behavior,* vol. 2 (Technical Reviews). Rockville, MD: U.S. Department of Health and Human Services.
Pearson, L. 1969. *Death and Dying: Current Issues in the Treatment of the Dying Person.* Cleveland: Cleveland Press of Western Reserve.
Pederson, P. B., et al. 1981. *Counseling Across Cultures.* Honolulu: University Press of Hawaii.
Percy, W. 1975. *Message in a Bottle.* New York: Farrar, Strauss & Giroux.
Perrine, L. 1962. *Poetry: Theory and Practice,* 3d ed. New York: Harcourt Brace.
______. 1969. *Sound and Sense: An Introduction to Poetry,* 3d ed. New York: Harcourt Brace.
______. 1978. *Literature: Structure, Sound and Sense.* New York: Harcourt Brace.
Pfeiffer, J., and Jones, J., eds. 1974. *A Sourcebook of Structured Experiences,* vols. 1–4. La Jolla, CA: University Association.
Phelps, I., and Dewine, S. 1976. *Interpersonal Communication Journal.* St. Paul, MN: West Publishing.

Pietropinto, A. 1975. "Poetry Therapy in Groups." In *Current Psychiatric Therapies*, vol. 15, ed. J. Masserman. New York: Grune.

Pilch, J. J. 1981. *Wellness: Your Invitation to Full Life*. Minneapolis: Winston Press.

Plessner, H. 1970. *Laughing and Crying: A Study of the Limits of Human Behavior*. Evanston, IL: Northwestern University Press.

Plutchik, R. 1980. "A Language for the Emotions." *Psychology Today* 13.9:68–78.

Ponzo, Z. 1974. "A Counselor and Change: Reminiscences and Resolutions." *Personnel and Guidance Journal* 53.1 (September):27–30.

Progoff, I. 1975. *At a Journal Workshop: The Basic Text and Guide for Using the Intensive Journal*. New York: Dialogue House Library.

Pullinger, W. F. 1958. "Remotivation." *Mental Hospitals* 9.16 (January).

______. 1960. "Remotivation." *American Journal of Nursing* 60.5 (May):682–685.

Quigley, P. 1981. *Those Were the Days: Life Review Therapy for Elderly Patients*. Buffalo, NY.

Rance, C., and Price, A. 1973. "Poetry as a Group Project." *American Journal of Occupational Therapy* 27.5:252–255.

Reik, T. 1949. *Listening with the Third Ear*. New York: Harcourt Brace.

Reiter, S. 1978a. "Poetry Therapy." *Art in Psychotherapy* 5.13–14.

______. 1978b. "Certification of the Poetry Therapist." *Association of Poetry Therapy News* 10.3.

Remacker, A. J., and Storch, E. T. 1982. *Actions Speak Louder: A Handbook of Non-verbal Techniques*, 3d ed. New York: Churchill Livingstone.

Reps, P. 1959. *Zen Telegrams*. Rutland, VT: Tuttle.

Reynolds, D., and Kalish, R. A. 1974. "The Social Ecology of Dying: Observations of Wards for the Terminally Ill." *Hospital and Community Psychiatry* 25.3 (March):147–159.

Rico, G. 1983. *Writing the Natural Way: Using Right Brain Techniques*. Los Angeles: J. P. Tarcher.

Ricoeur, P. 1974. "Psychiatry and Moral Values." In *The American Handbook of Psychiatry: The Foundations of Psychiatry*, vol. 1, 2d ed., ed. S. Arieti. New York: Basic Books.

______. 1978. "The Metaphorical Process as Cognition, Imagination, and Feeling." *Critical Inquiry* 5:143–159.

Riggs, C. W. 1971. *Bibliotherapy*. Newark: International Reading Association.

Rioch, M. J., et al. 1976. *Dialogue for the Therapists*. San Francisco: Jossey-Bass.

Roberts, C. 1982. "RET: Rational/Emotive Therapy—A Cognitive Behavior System." *Perspectives in Psychiatric Care* 20.3 (July-September):134–138.

Robinson, A. M. n.d. *Remotivation Techniques*, Smith Kline & French Laboratory Remotivation Project. Washington, DC: American Psychiatric Association.

Robinson, D. 1980. "A Bibliotherapy Program with Special Education Students." *Top of the News* (Winter):189–193.

Rogers, C. R. 1957. "Necessary and Sufficient Conditions of Therapeutic Personality Change." *Journal of Consulting Psychiatry* 21:95–103.

______. 1961. *On Becoming a Person*. New York: Houghton Mifflin.

______. 1966. "Client-centered Therapy." In *American Handbook of Psychiatry*, vol. 3, ed. S. Arieti, New York: Basic Books.

Rogers, C. R., and Dymond, R. F., eds. 1978. *Psychotherapy and Personality Change*. Chicago: University of Chicago Press.

Rogers, R. 1973. "The Metaphysics of Poetic Language: Modal Ambiguity." *International Journal of Psycho-Analytics* 54:61–74.

Rosenbaum, M., and Berger, M., eds. 1975. *Group Psychotherapy and Group Functions*, rev. ed., New York: Basic Books.

Rosenberg, M. 1979. *Conceiving the Self*. New York: Basic Books.

Rosenblatt, L. M. 1976. *Literature as Exploration*, 3d ed. New York: MLA.

______. 1978. *The Reader, the Text, the Poem: A Transactional Theory of the Literary Work*. Carbondale, IL: Southern Illinois University Press.

Ross, D.L.D. 1977. "Poetry Therapy Vs. Traditional Supportive Therapy: A Comparison of Group Process." Ph.D. thesis, Case Western Reserve.

Rossi, M. J. 1983. "Single-parent Families in Picture Books." *School Library Journal* 30.32–33.

Rothenberg, A. 1970. "Inspiration, Insight and the Creative Process in Poetry." *College English* 32:171–183.

______. 1972a. "Poetic Process and Psychotherapy." *Psychiatry* 35 (August):238–254.

______. 1972b. "Poetry in Therapy: Therapy in Poetry." *The Sciences* 12.4 (January-February):30–31.

______. 1979a. *The Emerging Goddess: The Creative Process in Art, Science, and Other Fields.* Chicago: University of Chicago Press.

______. 1979b. "Einstein's Creative Thinking and the General Theory of Creativity." *American Journal of Psychiatry* 136.1 (January):38–43.

______. 1979c. "Creative Contradictions." *Psychology Today* 13.1 (June):55–62.

Rothenberg, A., and Hausman, C., eds. 1976. *The Creativity Question.* Durham, NC: Duke University Press.

Rubin, R. 1974. "Prison Libraries: Focus on Service to the Ex-Advantaged." *Catholic Library World* 45 (April):438–440.

______. 1977. "The Use of Bibliotherapy in Corrections." In "Proceedings of the Bibliotherapy Round Table," ed. A. Hynes and K. Gorelick. Washington, DC.

______. 1978a. *Using Bibliotherapy: A Guide to Theory and Practice.* Phoenix, AZ: Oryx Press.

______. 1978b. *Bibliotherapy Sourcebook.* Phoenix, AZ: Oryx Press.

______. 1979. "Uses of Bibliotherapy in Response to the 1970s." *Library Trends* 28.2 (Fall):239–252.

______. 1982. "Reading Guidance and Bibliotherapy." In *The Service Imperative: Essays in Tribute to Margaret E. Monroe*, ed. G. Schalechter. Littleton, CO: Libraries Unlimited.

Rugg, H. O. 1963. *Imagination.* New York: Harper & Row.

Russell, A. E., and Russell, W. A. 1979. "Using Bibliotherapy with Emotionally Disturbed Children." *Teaching Exceptional Children* 11.4 (Summer):168–169.

Santayana, G. 1961. *The Sense of Beauty: Being the Outline of Aesthetic Theory.* New York: Collier.

Sargent, L. 1979. "Poetry in Therapy." *Social Work* 24.2 (March):157–159.

SASHA tapes (Self-automated Series on Helping Activities): Users manual and three tapes. Los Angeles: Interpersonal Research, UCLA Department of Psychology, UCLA extension.

Saul, S., and Saul, S. 1974. "Group Psychotherapy in a Proprietary Nursing Home." *Gerontologist* 14:446–450.

Schecter, R. L. 1983. *Poetry Therapy: A Therapeutic Tool and Healing Force.* New York: Julie Smith Association.

Schloss, G. A. 1976. *Psychopoetry.* New York: Grosset & Dunlap.

Schloss, G. A., and Grundy, D. E. 1978. "Action Techniques in Psychopoetry." In *Poetry in the Therapeutic Experience*, ed. A. Lerner. New York: Pergamon.

Schneck, J. M. 1945. "A Bibliography on Bibliotherapy and Hospital Library Activities." *Bulletin of the Medical Library Association* 33 (July):341–356.

______. 1950. "Bibliotherapy in Neuropsychiatry." In *Occupational Therapy: Principles and Practice*, ed. W. R. Dunton, Jr., and S. Licht. Springfield, IL: Thomas.

Schrank, F. A., and Engels, D. W. 1981. "Bibliotherapy as a Counseling Adjunct: Research Findings." *Personnel and Guidance Journal* 60.3 (November):143–147.

Schultheis, M. 1969. "A Study of the Effects of Selected Readings upon Children's Academic Performances and Social Adjustments." Ed.D. thesis, Ball State University, Muncie, IN.

______. 1972. *A Guidebook for Bibliotherapy.* Glenview, IL: Psychotechnics.

Sclabassi, S. H. 1973. "Literature as a Therapeutic Tool: A Review of the Literature on Bibliotherapy." *American Journal of Psychotherapy* 28 (January):70–77.

Senior Center Humanities Program. 1977. *Self-discovery Through the Humanities: Images of Aging in Literature.* Washington, DC: National Council on Aging.

Shave, D. 1974. *The Therapeutic Listener.* Huntington, NY: Krieger.

Sheiman, J. 1972. "The Case for 'Naturals' of Poetry Therapy" (paper presented at the Second Association of Poetry Therapy, Brooklyn, NY).

Shiryon, M. 1977a. "Poetry Therapy and the Theoretical and Practical Framework of Literatherapy." *Art Psychotherapy* 4.2:73–78.

______. 1977b. "Biblical Roots of Literatherapy." *Journal of Psychology and Judaism* 2.1 (Fall):3–11.

Shorr, J. E., et al. 1980. *Imagery: Its Many Dimensions and Applications.* New York: Plenum.
Shostrom, J. E., et al. 1980. *Actualizing Therapy: Foundations for a Scientific Ethic.* San Diego: EDITS.
Shrodes, C. 1949. "Bibliotherapy: A Theoretical and Clinical Experimental Study." Ph.D thesis, University of California, Berkeley.
Silverman, H. L. 1973. "Psychological Implications of Poetry Therapy." *Society and Culture* 4.2:215–228.
______. 1977. "Creativeness and Creativity in Poetry as a Therapeutic Process." *Art Psychotherapy* 4.1:19–28.
Silverstein, L. M., et al. 1977. *Consider the Alternative.* Minneapolis: Com Peare.
Simon, B. 1978. *Mind and Madness in Ancient Greece: The Classical Roots of Modern Psychiatry.* Ithaca, NY: Cornell University Press.
Singer, J. L. 1971. "The Vicissitudes of Imagery in Research and Clinical Use." *Continuing Psychoanalysis* 7.2 (Spring):163–180.
______. 1973. *The Child's World of Make-Believe.* New York: Academic Press.
______. 1975a. *The Inner World of Daydreaming.* New York: Harper & Row.
______. 1975b. "Boundary Management in Psychological Work with Groups." *Journal of Applied Behavioral Sciences* 11.2:137–176.
______. 1976. *Mind Play: The Creative Uses of Fantasy.* New York: Harper & Row.
Sohn, D. 1969. *Pictures for Writing.* New York: Bantam.
Sohngen, M., and Smith, R. J. 1978. "Images of Old Age in Poetry." *Gerontologist* 18.2:181–186.
Sorokin, P. 1950. "Love: Its Aspects, Production, Transformation, and Accumulation." In *Explorations in Altruistic Love and Behavior: A Symposium*, ed. P. Sorokin. Boston: Beacon (Kraus Reprint).
Starr, A. 1972. *The Dynamics of Creation.* New York: Atheneum.
Stephens, J. W. 1981. *A Practical Guide to the Use and Implementation of Bibliotherapy.* Great Neck, NY: Todd & Honeywell.
Strawson, P. F. 1970. "Imagination and Perception." In *Experience and Theory*, ed. L. Foster and J. W. Swanson. Amherst, MA: University of Massachusetts Press.
Strayhorn, J. M. 1983. "A Diagnostic Axis Relevant to Psychotherapy and Preventative Mental Health." *American Journal of Orthopsychiatry* 53.4 (October):677–696.
Sweeney, D. 1978. "Bibliotherapy and the Elderly." In *Bibliotherapy Sourcebook*, ed. R. Rubin. Phoenix, AZ: Oryx Press.
Swift, H. 1983. *AA and Bibliotherapy.* Center City, MN: Hazelden.
Taylor, C. W., ed. 1972. *Climate for Creativity: Report of the National Conference on Creativity.* New York: Pergamon.
Taylor, D. 1980. "Poetry from Non-Poets: A Simple Exercise in Creative Self-discovery." *Journal of Creative Behavior* 14.2:115–124.
Thomas, J., and Vaughan, M., eds. 1983. *Sharing Books with Young Children.* Minneapolis: T. S. Dennison.
Tolkien, J.R.R. 1974. "On Fairy Stories." In *Essays Presented to Charles Williams*, ed. C. S. Lewis. London: Oxford University Press.
Trotzer, J. P. 1977. *The Counselor and the Group: Integrating Theory, Training and Practice.* Monterey, CA: Brooks/Cole.
Turner, A. 1980. *Poets Teaching: The Creative Process.* New York: Longman.
Tuzil, T. J. 1978. "The Written Word and the Elderly: Adjunct to Treatment." *Journal of Gerontological Social Work* 1.1 (Fall):81–87.
Tyler, L. E. 1978. *Individuality: Human Possibilities and Personal Choice in the Psychological Development of Men and Women.* San Francisco: Jossey-Bass.
U.S. Congress, 94th Congress, 1970. An Act: *Title I—General Revision of Copyright Law* (P.L. 94-533. 90 STAT. 2541. 17 USC 107), p. ii.
Vaccaro, M. 1979. "Interfaces of Creativity in Therapy: A Mini-symposium." *Art Psychotherapy* 6.3:137–153.
Vail, P. 1981. *Clear and Lively Writing: Language Games and Activities for Everyone.* New York: Walker.
VanderPost, L. 1972. *A Story Like the Wind.* New York: Morrow.

Van Tichelt, R. A. 1977. "An Analysis of the Reading Process: Toward a Foundation in Bibliotherapy." Ph.D. thesis, California School of Professional Psychology.

Wadeson, H. 1981. "Self-exploration and Integration Through Poetry Writing." *Arts in Psychotherapy* 3, 3–4:225–236.

Wallick, M. M. 1980. "An Autistic Child and Books." *Top of the News* 37 (Fall):69–77.

Warner, L. 1980. "The Myth of Bibliotherapy." *School Library Journal* (October):107–111.

Waterman, A. S., et al. 1977. "The Role of Expressive Writing in Ego-Identity Formation." *Developmental Psychology* 13.3:286.

Watson, J. J. 1980. Bibliotherapy for Abused Children. *The School Counselor* (January):204–208.

Watzlawick, P. 1978. *The Language of Change: Elements of Therapeutic Communication.* New York: Basic Books.

Webb, E. J., et al. 1974. *Unobtrusive Measures: Nonreactive Research in the Social Sciences.* Chicago: Rand-McNally.

Wedl, L. 1983. "Bibliotherapy: A Counseling Tool to Promote Creative Aging in Older Persons." M.A. thesis, School of Applied Behavioral Sciences and Educational Leadership, Athens, Ohio University.

Weigart, E. 1960. "Loneliness and Trust: Basic Factors of Human Existence." *Psychiatry* 25:121–132.

———. 1961. "The Nature of Sympathy in the Art of Psychotherapy." *Psychiatry* 26.2:189–196.

Welch, J. G. 1982. *Topics for Getting in Touch: A Poetry Therapy Sourcebook.* Columbus, OH: Pudding Magazine.

Wiebe, K. F. 1979. *Good Times with Old Times: How to Write Your Memoirs.* Scottsdale, PA: Herald Press.

Wilson, J. B. 1979. *The Story Experience.* Metuchen, NJ: Scarecrow.

Wilson, L., and Goodman, R. 1980. "Establishing Civil Service Job Classifications for Creative Art Therapists in New York State." *American Journal of Art Therapy* 20.1:13–19.

Wolberg, L. R. 1967. *The Technique of Psychotherapy,* 2d ed. New York: Grune.

Yalom, I. 1975. *The Theory and Practice of Group Psychotherapy,* 2d rev. ed. New York: Basic Books.

———. 1980. *Existential Psychotherapy.* New York: Basic Books.

———. 1983. *Inpatient Group-Psychotherapy.* New York: Basic Books.

Yarrow, L. J. 1979. "Emotional Development." *American Psychologist* 34.10:951–957.

Zaccaria, J., Moses, H. A., and Hallowell, J. 1978. *Bibliotherapy in Rehabilitation: Educational and Mental Health Settings,* 2d ed. (1st ed. 1968). Champaign, IL: Stipes.

Zander, T. 1982. *Making Groups Effective* (Management Training and Development Series). San Francisco: Jossey-Bass.

Zwerling, I. 1979. "The Creative Art Therapies as 'Real Therapies.'" *Hospital and Community Psychiatry* 30.12 (December):841–844.

Bibliotherapeutic Materials Cited

Adoff, A., ed. 1969. *City in All Directions.* New York: Harper & Row.

______. 1973. *The Poetry of Black America.* New York: Harper & Row.

Aldis, D. 1936. "Hands," *Sung Under the Silver Umbrella.* New York: Macmillan.

______. 1936. "Feet." *Sung Under the Silver Umbrella.* New York: Macmillan.

Allen, S., comp. 1973. *Poems from Africa: Selected by Samuel Allen.* New York: Harper & Row.

Allen, T., ed. 1972. *Whispering Wind: Poetry by Young American Indians.* New York: Doubleday.

Antin, D. 1969. "Regarding a Door." *Some Haystacks Don't Even Have Needles,* ed. S. Dunning et al. Glenview, IL: Scott, Foresman.

Auden, W. H. 1945. "Musée des Beaux Arts." *The Collected Poetry of W. H. Auden.* New York: Random House.

Baker, K. W. 1968. "Days." *Time for Poetry,* 3d ed., ed. M. H. Arbuthnot and S. L. Root. Glenview, IL: Scott, Foresman.

Berne, E. 1964. *Games People Play.* New York: Ballantine.

Boyd, T., et al., eds. 1975a. "Loneliness." *Windows, Walls, Bridges.* Washington, DC: U.S. Government Printing Office.

______. 1975b. "To Those Who Understood Me." *Windows, Walls, Bridges.* Washington, DC: U.S. Government Printing Office.

Buber, M. 1975. *Tales of the Hassidim: The Later Masters,* trans. O. Marx. New York: Schocken.

Casey, B. 1969. "Look, See." *Look at All the People.* New York: Doubleday.

Cleaver, E. 1968. *Soul on Ice.* New York: McGraw-Hill.

Clifton, L. 1974. "I'm Running into a New Year." *An Ordinary Woman.* New York: Random House.

Conkling, H. 1968. "Butterfly." *Time for Poetry,* 3d ed., ed. M. H. Arbuthnot and S. L. Root. Glenview, IL: Scott, Foresman.

cummings, e. e. 1972. "maggie and milly and molly and may." *Complete Poems: 1913–1962.* New York: Harcourt Brace.

Cutler, I. 1981. "Alone." *Strictly Private,* ed. R. McGough. New York: Kestrel Books (Penguin).

De Regniers, B. S. 1968. "I Looked in the Mirror." *Piping Down the Valley Wild,* ed. N. Larrick. New York: Delacorte.

Der Hovanessian, D., and Morgassian, M., eds. 1978. *Anthology of Armenian Poetry.* New York: Columbia University Press.

Dickinson, E. 1963. "I'm Nobody, Who Are You?" *The Complete Poems of Emily Dickinson,* ed. T. H. Johnson. Boston: Little, Brown.

Donne, J. 1956. "A Valediction Forbidding Mourning." *Sound and Sense,* ed. L. Perrine. New York: Harcourt Brace.

Dunbar, P. 1967. "The Debt." *Kaleidoscopes*, ed. R. Hayden. New York: Harcourt Brace.
Dungan, A. 1974. "Prayer." *Atlantic Monthly* (March).
Eliot, T. S. 1952. "Four Quartets: East Coker, III." *The Complete Poems and Plays: 1909–1950*. New York: Harcourt Brace.
Evans, M. 1970. "The Silver Cell." *I Am a Black Woman*. New York: Morrow.
Farber, N. 1974. "I Know Daybreak." *Christian Science Monitor* (August 19).
Fisher, D. C. 1977. "The Heyday of the Blood." *Self-discovery Through the Humanities*. Washington, DC: National Council on Aging.
Fromm, E. 1956. *The Art of Loving*. New York: Harper & Row.
Frost, R. 1969. "Devotion." *The Poetry of Robert Frost*, ed. E. C. Lathem. New York: Holt, Rinehart & Winston.
______. 1969. "Lodged." *The Poetry of Robert Frost*, ed. E. C. Lathem. New York: Holt, Rinehart & Winston.
______. 1969. "The Mending Wall." *The Poetry of Robert Frost*, ed. E. C. Lathem. New York: Holt, Rinehart & Winston.
______. 1969. "Stopping by a Woods on a Snowy Evening." *The Poetry of Robert Frost*, ed. E. C. Lathem. New York: Holt, Rinehart & Winston.
George, J. C. 1972. *Julie of the Wolves*. New York: Harper & Row.
Gilpin, L. 1977. "Spring Cleaning." *Hocus-Pocus of the Universe*. New York: Doubleday.
Giovanni, N. 1977. "Legacies." *Crazy to Be Alive in Such a Strange World*, ed. N. Larrick. New York: Evans.
Haley, A. 1967. *Autobiography of Malcolm X*. New York: Dell.
Hoffer, E. 1975. "The Ordeal of Change." In *Windows, Walls, Bridges*, ed. T. Boyd et al. Washington, DC: U.S. Government Printing Office.
Hughes, L. 1949. "Mother to Son." *The Dream Keeper*. New York: Knopf.
______. 1961. *The Best of Simple*. New York: Hill & Wang.
Keillor, G. 1981. "My Stepmother, Myself." *Happy to Be Here*. New York: Penguin.
Larrick, N. 1968. *On City Streets*. New York: M. Evans.
Lawrence, D. H. 1958. "We Are Transmitters." *The Portable D. H. Lawrence*, ed. D. Trilling. New York: Viking.
Lennon, J. 1967. "When We're 64." *The Beatles/1962–1966*. Capitol Industries, Inc.
Lenski, L. 1968. "People." *On City Streets*, ed. N. Larrick. New York: Bantam.
Longfellow, H. W. 1962. "The Rainy Day." *McGuffey's Fifth Eclectic Reader: 1879 edition*. New York: Signet Classics.
Madgett, N. 1975. "Woman with Flower." *The Forerunners: Black Poets in America*, ed. Woodie King, Jr. Washington, DC: Howard University Press.
Marshall, H. L. 1976. "Grandma's Gumption." *Leave a Touch of Glory*. New York: Doubleday.
McGinnis, S. Z. "Love in a Plain Wrapper." *Rye Bread: Women Poets Rising*, ed. R. Tuthill and D. Kerr. Scope Publ.
Merriam, E. 1977. *Out Loud*. New York: Atheneum.
______. 1977. *It Doesn't Always Have to Rhyme*. New York: Atheneum.
Miles, Peggy Patrick. "Landscape: February." Used with permission of the author.
Mitchell, J. 1969. "I Think I Understand." *Clouds*. Reprise Records.
Morgan, E. 1981. "Hyena." *Strictly Private*, ed. R. McGough. New York: Kestrel Books (Penguin).
Morley, C. 1950. "Smells." *Living Poetry*, ed. H. J. McNeil and D. S. Zimmer. New York: Globe Books.
Nathan, R. 1955. "I Ride the Great Black Horses of My Heart." *Modern American Poetry: Modern British Poetry*, ed. L. Untremeyer. New York: Harcourt Brace.
Park, F. 1966. "A Sad Song About Greenwich Village." *On City Streets*, ed. N. Larrick. New York: Bantam.
Po Chu-I. 1970. "Pruning Trees." *A Flock of Words*, ed. D. MacKay. New York: Harcourt Brace.
Poe, E. A. 1957. "Bells." *Favorite Poems Old and New*, ed. H. Ferris. New York: Doubleday.
Robinson, E. A. 1955. "Richard Cory." *Modern American Poetry: Modern British Poetry*, ed. L. Untermeyer. New York: Harcourt Brace.
Sandburg, C. 1974. "Soup." *Take Hold!* ed. L. B. Hopkins. Nashville, TN: Nelson.
Solzhenitsyn, A. 1967. *Cancer Ward*, trans. T. P. Whitney. New York: Bantam.

Southey, R. 1962. "The Cataract of Lodore." *McGuffey's Fifth Ecletic Reader: 1879 Edition.* New York: Signet Classics.

Stevens, C. n.d. "I'm on the Road to Find Out." *Tea for the Tillerman.* A and M Records.

Thomas, Dylan. 1963. "Do Not Go Gentle into that Good Night." *Mentor Book of Major British Poets,* ed. O. Williams. New York: Mentor.

Thurber, James. 1952. "The Courtship of Arthur and Al." *Fables for Our Times.* New York: Harper & Row.

Updike, J. 1969. "Ex-Basketball Player." *Some Haystacks Don't Even Have Any Needles,* ed. Stephen Dunning et al. Glenview, IL: Scott, Foresman.

Walker, A. 1983. "In Search of My Mother's Garden." *In Search of Our Mothers' Gardens.* New York: Harcourt Brace.

Wilkinson, Betty. 1970. "Why Do They?" *I Heard a Scream in the Streets,* ed. N. Larrick. New York: Evans.

Willette, F. H. 1969. *Shadows and Light.* St. Cloud, MN: North Star Press.

Worth, V. 1972. *Small poems, More Small Poems.* New York: Farrar, Strauss & Giroux.

Yeats, W. B. 1955. "Among School Children." *Modern American Poetry: Modern British Poetry,* ed. L. Untermeyer. New York: Harcourt Brace.

Index

For Product Safety Concerns and Information please contact our EU representative GPSR@taylorandfrancis.com Taylor & Francis Verlag GmbH, Kaufingerstraße 24, 80331 München, Germany

Batch number: 10726009

Printed by Printforce, the Netherlands